Yogic Management
of Cancer

With kind regards, ॐ and prem

Yogic Management of Cancer

Dr Swami Nirmalananda

Yoga Publications Trust, Munger, Bihar, India

Published by Yoga Publications Trust
    First edition 2009

ISBN: 978-81-86336-81-6

Publisher and distributor: Yoga Publications Trust, Ganga Darshan, Munger, Bihar, India.

Website: www.biharyoga.net
        www.rikhiapeeth.net

Printed at Thomson Press (India) Limited, New Delhi, 110001

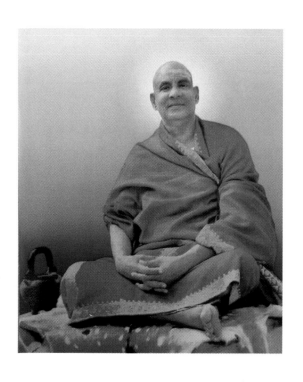

Dedication

*In humility we offer this dedication to
Swami Sivananda Saraswati, who initiated
Swami Satyananda Saraswati into the secrets of yoga.*

Contents

Contents

Introduction

Nothing needs to be feared; it just needs to be understood clearly. As the wise saying goes, "the only thing to fear is fear itself." When we are not fully aware of what are we dealing with, we cannot come to any definite plan of action. This indecisiveness leads to feelings of insecurity and fear. Even if a situation or person is friendly and beneficial, doubt can lurk in the mind until we have understanding. The moment we know the situation or person to our satisfaction, our confidence returns with the ability to act appropriately and with a positive outcome. This book is an attempt to make the unknown facts about cancer more understandable and also to help outline a coping strategy using yoga. In this way we can move beyond fear and into productive action.

This book has three objectives. The first objective is to understand cancer clearly by investigating the facts and removing the misconceptions about cancer. This is the area of science. The author has also introduced a view that every disease state, including cancer, manifests in the body when the inherent qualities of living beings called *gunas* become grossly imbalanced.

The second objective is to understand ourselves and our inherent resources. We should understand our real needs as well as the strengths we have that can be utilized to fulfil these needs and how best to proceed on this path. We should also know the limitations we have that can prevent us fulfilling these needs and know how to manage those limitations. We should try to identify which skills or qualities we need to cultivate and how to do this. This is the area of yoga.

Once we know the nature of cancer, the stressor, and of 'I', the stressed, we can work out a winning and coping strategy. The third objective, therefore, is to identify and implement the chosen coping methods to overcome the crisis or at least to manage it adequately. This area covers the fields of science and yoga together.

Yogic teaching counsels that one should fight against the adverse situation in the best way and as far as possible, but one must also have the courage to accept whatever outcome eventuates, favourable or not, with complete dignity, making the best of that outcome. Yoga provides the wisdom to know when and how much to fight, and when and how to accept.

Yoga practices are not symptom specific. Prescriptions such as 'for coughing asana A will help, for constipation practice B will help and practice C is a cure for all – from cold to cancer' do not hold true. Yoga is a holistic science. A balanced set of practices done regularly with a positive and mature attitude towards life can remedy most general problems. One or two practices can then be added or removed to cater to the current specific issue.

The techniques of the yoga practices are given separately in the practice section after the relevant chapter. Only very simple practices have been chosen for the safety of the practitioner. The book is not intended to be a complete guide for a cancer patient. The guidance of a teacher is essential. The subject of yoga is so vast that no book can be a complete authority. It is not possible to cover every practice mentioned in the text, only some practices that are particularly useful to cancer patients are included. For a broader coverage refer to the relevant publications of Yoga Publications Trust, Munger, India. References are given where relevant.

This book does not offer yoga as a cure for cancer or as a miracle, but acknowledges that the possibility is there. What yoga does offer is a solid and reliable support to lean on. It helps one connect to the source of inner strength and become self-reliant. It trains one to deal with the issues of life as they arise.

The need for yoga, the need to connect to the inner self, is the same in a sick or a healthy person. Some people are more sensitive to this need and some are less so. When cancer or any other serious difficulty obstructs the free flow of life, the need for this inner connection becomes evident and pressing. So although this book is written for people with cancer, it is equally useful for any seriously ill person and also for those without any sickness, who are eager to explore the benefits of yoga.

This book is based on the teachings of Swami Satyananda Saraswati and Swami Niranjanananda Saraswati. Just as a mirror can only reflect what is in front of it and an audio device can only emit the words recorded on it, so too the mind of a disciple can only reflect what has been engraved on it by the guru.

1: Understanding Cancer

1

Health and Disease

Health

The Sanskrit word for health is very apt. It defines good health in just one word – *swastha*. This word is made up of *swa*, meaning 'the self', and *stha*, meaning 'to be established in'. One whose consciousness is established in the self is the possessor of good health. In order to peacefully establish awareness in one's inner core, or centre, there should be no disturbances in the bodily functions, mental faculties, emotions or interactions with the external world and there should be perfect contentment with one's life situation. This short definition of health fulfils all the criteria of the modern definition of good health given by the World Health Organization (WHO): "Good health is a sense of wellbeing at physical, psychological, emotional, social and spiritual levels."

The yogic view is exactly the same. In yoga, good health means harmony in all the five *koshas* or bodies: *annamaya kosha* (physical body), *pranamaya kosha* (energy body), *manomaya kosha* (mental body), *vijnanamaya kosha* (wisdom or intuitive body) and *anandamaya kosha* (bliss body). The koshas are explored in greater detail in chapter 5.

Ayurveda, the vedic science of health, considers health to be a state where all three *doshas* (biological humours) of the body: *vata* (wind, gas), *pitta* (bile) and *kapha* (mucus, phlegm), are well balanced and in harmony. *Sushruta Samhita* (15:44)

7

defines a swastha (a person in good health) as one whose doshas, somatic and psychic humours, are in a state of equilibrium, the digestive capacity is uniformly balanced, the fundamental tissues of the body and waste excretion are functioning normally, and the soul, cognitive organs and mind are in a lucid state.

The concept of guna

Gunas are the inherent qualities that determine the state of our mind and motivate our behaviour. They influence our thought processes, our preferences, the strength of our will, and hence the way we live our lives. There are three gunas: sattwa, rajas and tamas. *Sattwa guna* is characterized by balance and wisdom, *rajas* by activity and *tamas* by inertia and ignorance.

The constantly changing gunas influence the state of our health. Sattwa guna is responsible for positive states of mind and balanced body systems and is conducive to good health. Rajas guna causes over-stimulation of the mind and body systems, and according to yoga is implicated in stress-induced diseases like hypertension, diabetes and acidity. Similarly, tamas guna is associated with negative states of mind and weak body systems, leading to problems like cancer, auto-immune disorders, degenerative disorders and depression. Health depends upon the way we live our life. If we do not take the rudder of the boat of our lives in our hands consciously and activate the required guna, the boat will sail in any direction spontaneously under the influence of the predominant guna at that moment, thereby inviting various diseases. This topic is dealt with in greater detail in chapter 4.

The science of yoga is about re-establishing the dormant link between the individual and his inner self. This activates sattwa guna. In order to establish this link the bodily functions, mental faculties, emotions and social interactions need to be balanced through yogic practices. The reverse is equally true. As an individual comes closer to his real self, his bodily functions, mental faculties, emotions and social interactions become balanced as the disturbances are sorted out. The key is a feeling of contentment and inner joy. This restores the balance. The positive energy of this state rushes to the area where there is a weakness, whether it be in an organ, the mind or the emotions, and mends it. As one starts coming closer to oneself, glimpses of this feeling are experienced.

Medical science now accepts that there are different stages of disturbances or imbalances before the state of health changes into a manifest disease. It is much easier to stay healthy than to change the state of disease into good health. Milder disturbances can be restored comparatively easily, but even the most stubborn of diseases can yield to the power of inner will. The quality of life, whether in health or in sickness, is completely in our own hands. So, wherever one is stationed, there the journey must begin. Once the journey begins, it definitely takes us towards the destination.

Steps to good health
The body and mind's normal nature is to stay healthy. They are resourceful enough to mend themselves unless provoked too adversely. The only exception to this rule is the effect of ageing, as the body's regenerative powers decrease with age. Usually it is our lifestyle that tips the balance of health. There are eight very simple rules that maintain good health or re-establish it when it is disturbed. In their absence, no therapy can be substantially effective.

1. Regularity in daily living: Normal daily activities like waking, bowel movements, taking a shower, eating, sleeping etc. should happen at their regular time. If we look to the laws of nature, we find regularity everywhere, from sunrise to sunset, from the waxing to the waning of the moon, from high tide to low tide, from season to season. This allows law and order to prevail in nature and for life to go on easily and to flourish. If there is irregularity and chaos, nature cannot survive or flourish. Similarly, if there is irregularity in one's life, one cannot stay healthy and grow.

2. Moderation in activities: Every activity needs to be performed in moderation. This regulation of behaviour is known as *samyam*. Avoid too much or too little of any activity. For example, a student may neglect their studies during the whole academic term and then study for fifteen hours a day during exams; an executive spending over twelve hours in the office may still bring work home on a regular basis and find no time for family matters; a teenager may spend long hours talking on the phone or chatting on the internet. All good things or activities are only good when limited to the appropriate quantity. Too much or too little of anything is harmful. Yoga always advocates the middle path.

3. Balance between physical and mental activity: Every person, of any age, must have eight hours of productive work daily, seven days a week. Of these eight hours at least two hours should be spent in hard physical work and two hours in intellectual work. This will keep both the body and mind healthy and sharp. If either aspect is neglected, its faculties degenerate.

4. Simple nourishing diet: The diet should be balanced in all nutrients and essential elements, easy to digest, clean, fresh and seasonal, moderate in quantity and consumed while in a positive frame of mind. It is said that what you eat, so you become. Food is directly responsible for the state of the body. The type of food consumed influences the type of thoughts crossing the mind.

5. Being in alignment with nature:

a) The way of living should be appropriate for the place and time. For example, in a cold country or in windy weather the body should be protected with adequate clothing, while in hot weather, cooling food items need to be consumed; at sunrise the body should be active and after sunset gradually withdrawn from activity. A lifestyle that follows the natural cycles and rhythms allows one to draw strength from nature, to reap the beneficial effects of the natural environment and also to be protected from the harmful ones.

b) Spending time enjoying the beauty and wonders of nature from time to time is energizing, de-stressing and helps create a positive frame of mind.

6. Being in good company: Known as *satsang*, this means spending time regularly in the company of wise and pure hearted people, studying inspiring books or other sources of information and participating in uplifting activities. These help us imbibe good concepts and activate our dormant positive qualities.

7. Self-observation and analysis: Known as *swadhyaya*, this means observing one's own behaviour, words and thoughts on a daily basis or from moment to moment, and trying to bring about any necessary changes that will enable the fulfilment of our goal in life. Through this exercise transformation occurs – the person who practises swadhyaya becomes a better person. This process goes on in every moment of the aspirant's life.

8. Expanding the horizon of the mind beyond 'I-mine': Known as *seva* or service, this means thinking, feeling and working not only for oneself or people dear to oneself but also for unknown people, without expectation of any return. Seva helps us to experience peace, contentment and joy.

Fig. 1.1: Eight Steps to Good Health

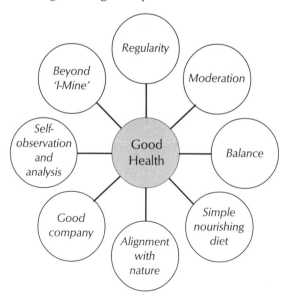

Disease

The absence of good health is ill health. Disease, dis+ease, is a state of ill health where the symptoms start manifesting at the level of the body and/or mind. On the long road originating at 'good health' and culminating at 'disease', there are many stations. The very first station is 'loss of inner peace and contentment'. The second station is 'loss of discrimination and inability to hear the inner guiding voice'. Subsequently passing through many alternative routes and intervening stations come the stations of 'loss of sense of wellbeing', 'low energy states and fatigue', 'poor appetite', 'inability to get adequate sleep', etc. before the destination of 'disease' is finally arrived at.

The state of disease itself can be classified into four stages. In the first or psychological stage, the symptoms are only at the level of the mind. The second stage is psychosomatic, where mental symptoms percolate into the body occasionally. In the third or somatic stage, the physical symptoms outweigh the mental symptoms, but the disturbance in the body is reversible. In the final organic stage there are irreversible structural changes in the body, making the disease a permanent guest.

Fig. 1.2: Development of Disease

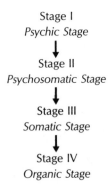

Stage I
Psychic Stage
↓
Stage II
Psychosomatic Stage
↓
Stage III
Somatic Stage
↓
Stage IV
Organic Stage

Drs Kothari and Mehta[1] classify diseases into two groups – interactional and intrinsic. Interactional diseases arise as a consequence of the unfavourable interaction between a human being and his environment. They are nutritive (e.g. iron deficiency anaemia), microbial (e.g. any infection), mechanical (e.g. fracture, heat stroke) or allergic (e.g. hay fever, allergic dermatitis). All interactional diseases lend themselves to control or prevention. Intrinsic diseases are programmed in one way or another into a human being's growth from womb to tomb. Birth defects or metabolic diseases that are likely to be genetically based (like high blood pressure, over-acidity of the stomach, autoimmune diseases), benign tumours and cancer are some examples of intrinsic diseases. It is not possible to find a definite cause for them, only contributing factors. They cannot be completely controlled or prevented, but can be managed to a smaller or greater extent.

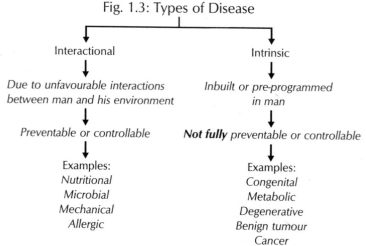

Fig. 1.3: Types of Disease

Factors contributing to ill health

- Inconsistency over a considerable period in observing the 'eight steps to good health'
- Ageing process or other causes of wear and tear
- Changes in environment, including natural and man-made calamities
- Fructification of past karma (refer to chapter 3).

Only the first factor is in the hands of the individual; the other three are more or less beyond individual control. One can only partly influence them.

2

Understanding Cancer

What is cancer?

A collection of abnormal cells is called a tumour. A tumour can be either malignant, if the cells are cancerous, or benign, if the constituent cells are not cancerous. Cancer is a disease of cells characterized by genetic mutation, abnormal cells, unrestrained cell production, lack of cell maturation (differentiation), loss of normal cellular function, invasive behaviour (invasion of normal neighbouring tissue) and often metastasis (spread of the cancer via lymphatic and/or blood flow to distant organs).

Fig. 2.1: Characteristics of a Cancer Cell

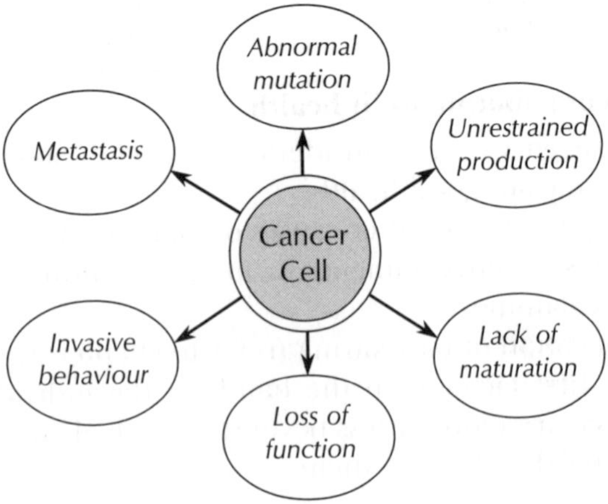

Cancer attacks many forms of life with equally devastating force – fish, birds and animals as well as humans. The cancer cells are not regulated by the normal biochemical and physical forces of the body. They behave like an unregulated entity. For some reason the cell's genetic material (DNA) undergoes irreversible structural change (mutation). As a result, the cell loses its normal function and starts behaving erratically. It starts growing and multiplying very rapidly. It compresses the surrounding normal cells and competes very aggressively with them for nutrients and space. Eventually it invades the normal surrounding tissue. It not only affects the neighbouring tissues, but also spreads to distant organs by moving through the lymphatic system and the blood stream or through body cavities, adversely affecting these distant organs.

One-third of all cancers are preventable, a further one third, if diagnosed sufficiently early, are potentially curable, and appropriate palliative care of the remaining one-third can bring about substantial improvements in the quality of life.[2] Although it is generally difficult to detect cancer at an early, curable stage, the most important step in our fight against cancer remains its prevention and early detection.

The cancer is named after the area of origin in the body, for example, lung cancer, brain cancer, breast cancer. When it spreads to distant organs, it is still identified as cancer of the original organ. For example, when a breast cancer spreads to the bones, it is called breast cancer with secondary deposits, or metastases, in the bone, rather than being called bone cancer. Occasionally the primary (original) site of cancer is unknown and only the metastasis is diagnosed.

Any area in the body can develop cancer. Worldwide, deaths due to cancer are most commonly caused by lung, stomach, liver, bowel, oesophagus and prostate cancers among men; and breast, lung, stomach, colorectal and cervical cancers among women. However, the incidence of cancer differs between countries. For example, stomach cancer is rare in the USA and common in Japan. Cervical cancer is uncommon in the West, but a leading cause of cancer-related death in

India. It should be noted that the majority of cancer-related deaths occur in low- and middle-income countries. The stressors and diet associated with western lifestyle render the population of developed countries more susceptible to the development of cancer. However, the number of people actually developing and dying of cancer is much greater in developing countries, for several reasons. Firstly, the population in low/middle income countries is much larger. Secondly, their life expectancy is gradually improving, increasing the incidence of cancer. Thirdly, they are less aware of preventive and early detection measures. Fourthly, some of their habits, such as chewing tobacco, unsafe sex, bearing many children etc., make them highly susceptible to certain cancers, like oropharyngeal and cervical cancer. Lastly, they have limited resources for cancer therapy. So the total number of deaths is much higher, but the overall percentage is still lower than in developed countries.[3]

The stages of cancer describe the extent of the cancerous growth, including the size of the primary tumour, the level of spread to the lymph nodes and the presence or absence of metastasis. Identifying the stage of cancer is often used to establish the prognosis and decide the treatment. Some cancers have a pre-cancerous stage. At this stage they are generally completely reversible. Dysplasia of the cervix and some types of leukoplakia of the oral cavity are the most commonly found pre-cancerous diseases. More details can be found in chapter 8.

DEVELOPMENT OF CANCER

Role of genes

The genetic material in the nucleus of a cell carries all the information for the functioning of that cell. In cancer these genes undergo change (mutation) and guide the cell into abnormal behaviour. There are three types of genes involved in cell growth. Their mutations can lead to cancer (see Fig. 2.2).

16

1. Proto-oncogenes are normal genes that regulate normal growth of cells. When they mutate into oncogenes and fail to function properly, abnormal cancer cells can begin to grow. More than thirty oncogenes have been identified. They can be tumour specific; with activation of a particular oncogene causing a particular cancer.
2. Tumour suppressor genes are normal genes that allow the body to recognize the abnormal growth of damaged or cancerous cells. They interrupt abnormal cell growth. When tumour suppressor genes mutate, this ability is lost and cancerous cells are more likely to be allowed to grow. The most important tumour suppressor gene known so far is p53. It suppresses uncontrolled proliferation of the cell as well as triggering apoptosis (programmed cell death) in cancerous cells. It is found to be mutated in about 50 percent of human cancers. Solar radiation, particularly ultraviolet, induces permanent mutation in p53, often leading to skin cancer.
3. Mutations of 'mismatch repair genes' are implicated in certain cancers. Normally, mismatch repair genes detect and correct DNA abnormalities arising during DNA replication. However, when these genes mutate, it is thought to be more likely that abnormal DNA will go undetected so abnormal cells will continue to survive and reproduce. Their role in cancer is controversial.

A series of mutations over a period of time is needed before a cell turns cancerous. This is possibly the reason for cancer being more common in old age. Mutation can occur without any identifiable cause, or can be due to exposure to mutagenic (mutation-causing) substances. Various agents that facilitate or induce the process of mutation have been identified and new ones continue to be recognized. Cancer-causing agents are known as carcinogens.

Carcinogens can be physical, such as radiation, including sunlight; chemical, such as tobacco and free oxygen radicals; or biological, such as hepatitis B virus and human papilloma virus (HPV). Additionally, from a yogic point of view, suppressed emotions, vicious patterns of thinking and negative emotions, including guilt, frustration, revenge and sadness are also injurious. A yogic lifestyle and attitude towards life provide an environment with minimum carcinogens. By minimizing our exposure to these carcinogens, we try to minimize the occurrence, growth or recurrence of cancer. However, minimum or no exposure to carcinogens does not guarantee freedom from cancer because, as explained earlier, the process of mutation can occur without any identifiable precipitant.

Fig. 2.2: Genetic Basis of Genesis of Cancer

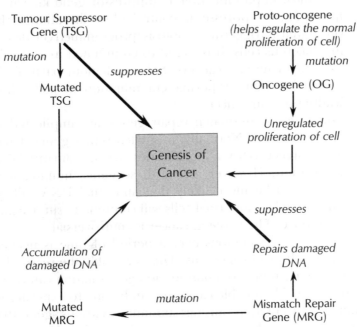

Role of the immune system

Under normal circumstances the immune system senses the abnormally behaving cells and tries to destroy them. The immune system operates through two main modes. The first is antibody-mediated (humoral) immunity. In this form of immunity, antibodies against the harmful substances are

18

produced. In a second form of immunity, known as cell mediated immunity, immune system cells are induced to destroy harmful substances by doing such things as physically engulfing the harmful substance or producing specific defensive chemicals (see Fig. 2.3). When the immune system fails, then cancer gains the upper hand and a tumour can develop. The malignant transformation of a cell is probably not a critical event in the development of cancer. Rather, it is the body's inability to destroy the newly formed cancerous cells when they are few in number that leads to the manifestation of cancer.

Under-nutrition, old age, HIV infection, some forms of drug abuse and chronic stress are some of the common causes of suppression of the immune system. Lack of protein and deficiencies of pyridoxine, folic acid, zinc and vitamins A, C and E can impair immune responses. Severe unaccustomed exercise induces stress and can diminish immune responses temporarily. The immune system may be suppressed by the long term use of corticosteroids and certain other therapeutic drugs.

Emotional states of mind affect the autonomic nervous system and endocrine system (see chapter 3 for more details), which in turn strongly influence the functioning of the immune system. Many studies have demonstrated that a reduction in immunity is associated with some types of stress (Segerstrom, 2004).[4] It is clear that the state of mind can play a major role in the efficiency of the immune system. Yoga helps us to understand the workings of our mind and provides techniques to help manage it efficiently. Regular practice and a yogic lifestyle helps to boost our immune system by releasing stress and creating a positive and stable frame of mind.

From a yogic viewpoint, a polluted environment puts a strain on the immune system by overloading it. A clean environment is highly charged with energy *(prana)* and negative ions that boost the immune system. The mind also spontaneously shifts into a happy, peaceful state in a clean environment, thus further strengthening the immune system.

19

Fig. 2.3: Immune System and its Basic Role in Cancer

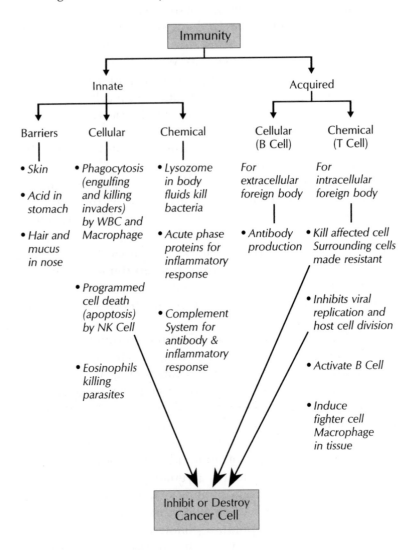

Fig. 2.4: Simplified Presentation of Development of Cancer

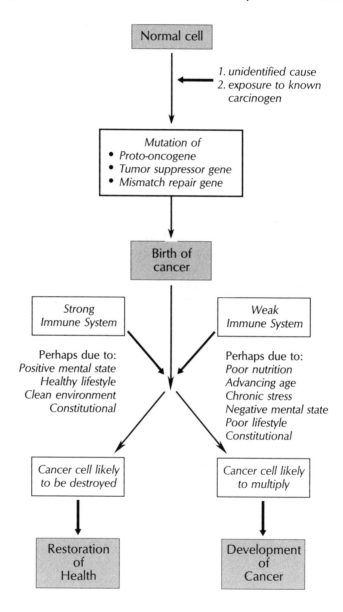

Types of cancer

Based on the original cell type, most of the human cancers are classified into the following types:

1. *Carcinoma*: arising from tissue called epithelial tissue. This tissue covers internal and external surfaces of the body (for example, it includes the skin and the lining of the digestive tract.) Carcinomas comprise more than 80% of human cancers. They can be further subdivided into squamous cell carcinoma, basal cell carcinoma and glandular cell or adeno-carcinoma. Includes most types of bowel, lung and breast cancer.

2. *Sarcoma*: arising from connective tissue such as bone, cartilage, fat, muscle etc.

3. *Other*: examples include leukaemia (blood cancers), lymphoma (lymphatic tissue cancers) and less common tumours arising from nerve cells.

Common warning symptoms of cancer

In its early stages, cancer is often a silent disease. Having said this, there are some symptoms of cancer that do occur: these are represented by a mnemonic CAUTION.

C Change in bowel or bladder habit

A Abnormal bleeding or discharge from any site

U Ulcer (sore) that does not heal; Unexplained weight loss or anaemia

T Thickening or lump anywhere

I Indigestion or difficulty in swallowing

O Obvious change in a wart or mole

N Nagging cough or persistent change in voice.

(It is important to remember that these symptoms frequently occur and do *not* represent cancer.)

3

Causes of Cancer

Our knowledge of cancer dates back to the earliest days of civilization. Evidence of cancer has been found in prehistoric animals and humans. Sushruta, the ayurvedic expert, mentions cancer in his *Sushruta Samhita*, written before 600 BC.

No real cause

There is no known single cause responsible for cancer. Medical science has identified many factors, known as carcinogens, that singly or in a group contribute to the formation of cancer. Carcinogens can damage DNA, causing the mutation of genes which ultimately leads to cancer. There can be a long latent period, a time gap of many years between exposure to the causative or contributing factor and the actual manifestation of the disease.

Cancer arises principally as a consequence of the conditions of life – namely, environmental factors (including exposure to carcinogens), biological factors, individual lifestyle or habits (such as tobacco use) and from a yogic viewpoint, the state of mind. But even if all these factors are healthy, there is no guarantee that cancer will not arise, as already explained in chapter 2. Cancer can be found in very young children, in animals and even in plants, albeit via different mechanisms. Cancer existed in previous millennia in spite of minimum pollution and simple lifestyles. Cancer, therefore, appears to be a condition intrinsic to life. While factors making cancer more likely have been identified, so far it has not been possible to find a definite cause for cancer, nor to completely control or prevent it.

Certain substances produced by the body, called free radicals, are inevitable consequences of necessary cellular metabolism. However, they probably also contribute to the process of mutation of genetic material. For this reason these free radicals, or oxidants, are sometimes called endogenous mutagens. These oxidants accumulate in the body and are thought to contribute to the process of ageing as well as the genesis of cancer. Some chemicals known as antioxidants counteract the effects of oxidants and so provide some protection. They are found in our diet or can be taken as a dietary supplement. More information can be found in chapter 9.

Let us now consider various factors that may increase the risk of cancer formation.

Table 3.1: Cancer: Key Risk Factors

Lifestyle Factors	
Tobacco	*Both active and passive smoking, and chewing*
Alcohol	
Dietary excesses	*Excess fats* *Heterocyclic amines* *Acrylamide*
Obesity	
Malnutrition	*Deficient fibre* *Possibly deficiencies of antioxidant micro-nutrients such as certain vitamins, and minerals like magnesium & selenium*
Food chemicals	*See Table 3.2*
Occupational materials	*Asbestos, benzene, benzedrine and formaldehyde (used in industrial manufacture), vinyl chloride (plastic manufacture)*

Environmental Factors	
Sunlight	*Excess sunlight (UV radiation)*
Ionizing radiation	*X-rays, nuclear fallout*
Pollution	*Pesticides, metals (arsenic, lead and others)*

Biological Factors	
Age	*Advancing age*
Repeated trauma	*For example, long term scratching of a spot so that it cannot heal can lead to the site transforming into certain types of skin cancer*
Pharmaceutical drugs	*Hormone replacement therapy may increase the risk of some cancers; some drugs used to treat cancer are associated with a risk of the development of cancer in other parts of the body*
Viruses and bacteria	*Human papilloma virus, hepatitis B and C virus, human immunodeficiency virus, Helicobacter pylori*
Psychological influences	*Some studies show suppression of negative emotions and a feeling of helplessness are linked to the spread and growth of cancer. According to studies so far, there is a stronger association between psychological stress and the spread of cancer than the initial development of cancer[5, 6]*
Genetics	*Some cancers are linked to inherited genetic mutations. Most cancers do not run in families*

Table 3.2: Carcinogens Possibly Present in Food

Possible Food Carcinogens *	
Alcohol	
Acrylamide:	*found in potato chips that have been deep fried and some other foods cooked at particularly high temperatures*
Fat:	*through obesity link*
Fish:	*large predatory fish such as shark may contain carcinogens*
Processed meats:	*possibly due to nitrites*
Heterocyclic amines:	*found in meat, especially when it is cooked at very high temperatures such as when fried or barbecued*
Pesticides and herbicides:	*can be carcinogenic. Vegetables and fruits sometimes contain low levels of these chemicals. At present there is no solid evidence linking cancer in humans with exposure to pesticides at the levels found in fruit and vegetables*
Pickled and salt-preserved foods:	*stomach, nasopharyngeal and throat cancers*
Soy:	*high levels could increase risk of estrogen-responsive cancers such as breast and uterine*
Sugar:	*through obesity link*
Trans-saturated fats:	*possible link. All fats have a link with obesity*
Vitamin A:	*excessive doses (as in too many supplements) may increase lung cancer risk.*

*Information from American Cancer Society and (US) National Cancer Institute.

The list is long and one can try to eliminate or minimize as many factors as possible. Developing a little awareness and simplicity in life can have positive effects.

PSYCHOLOGICAL FACTORS

Until recently medical science has restricted its extensive research to the external causative factors for cancer. But there is also a whole realm of the internal world, i.e. the mind and its activities, that according to yoga can influence the cancer process. The mind is an extremely powerful force that can create a state of health or destroy it. Academic research on mind potentiality and influence has only started recently.

Workings of the mind

Our five senses constantly take in information from the external world. The information is then sent to the brain and recognized by the mind. According to yoga the mind is functionally divided into four components: *manas*, the lower mind, *chitta*, the memory principle, *ahamkara*, the I-principle or self identity, and *buddhi*, the higher intellect.

Fig. 3.1: Functioning of Mind

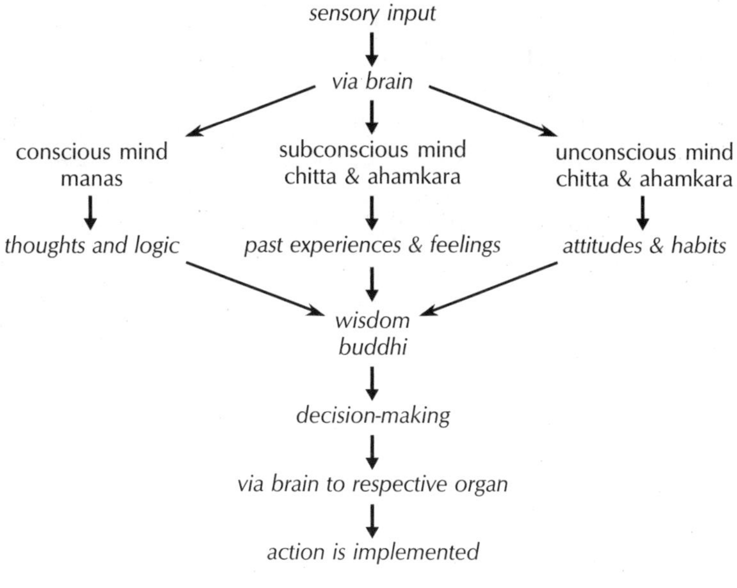

sensory input
↓
via brain
↓

conscious mind   subconscious mind   unconscious mind
manas   chitta & ahamkara   chitta & ahamkara
↓   ↓   ↓
thoughts and logic   past experiences & feelings   attitudes & habits

wisdom
buddhi
↓
decision-making
↓
via brain to respective organ
↓
action is implemented

When new information is received by the mind, it is sent to the first three components. Manas evaluates it using logic, chitta evaluates it in the light of past experience, and ahamkara evaluates it from the point of 'I and mine', 'What will the effect be on me?' The original information along with the perspective of the three faculties is passed on to buddhi. Buddhi uses its wisdom and discriminative skills to decide on the appropriate action to take in response to the information received. This decision is conveyed to the relevant organ of action via the brain and relevant nerves. The action is then carried out.

Patanjali's *Yoga Sutras* aptly describe the workings of the mind. It says an *iccha* (conscious or expressed desire) directs one's action. The force of desire compels one to act in a particular way. An action may be a physical act or a mental act (thought). The act of doing something creates an experience, good or bad. Also, the action bears a fruit (result). The result of the action also generates an experience, good or bad. Experience creates a *samskara* (impression in the deeper layers of the mind in the form of an archetype). All experiences teach us something. This learning is stored in chitta (memory) and is called a 'samskara'. A samskara creates a *vasana* (subtle or dormant desire). It can stay dormant for any length of time, from a second to many lives. The person will not be aware of its existence. At a certain time, triggered by a stimulating event, the vasana is converted into iccha, conscious desire. And thus the cycle continues endlessly.

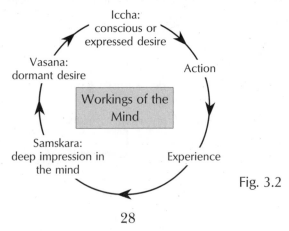

Fig. 3.2

28

A constructive, positive and creative desire leads to a positive cycle of events and a positive state of health while a negative, destructive desire leads to a negative cycle of events and a state of disease. Yoga shows the way to end this negative cycle or to convert it into a positive one. Depending on the personality and nature of the individual, this transformation can happen either through the meditative practices of raja yoga, the self-analytical practices of jnana yoga, the self-surrender practices of bhakti yoga, or the selfless service of karma yoga. Chapter 7 gives details of these different aspects of yoga.

By developing the awareness component of yoga practices, we learn to 'catch' the negative desire, action or experience while it is actually happening. This then enables us to withdraw at that moment, and in this way short-circuit the negative cycle. If the cycle has already reached the samskara stage, then generally it has to be lived through. When it next reaches the desire-action stage, the opportunity is there to rectify it. Sometimes, however, in altered states of consciousness during yoga practice, the samskara may involuntarily come to the surface in the form of a thought or image. When this happens, the samskara can be dealt with appropriately and thus exhausted, ending the cycle. Similarly, the positive cycles may be enhanced or reinforced when so required, by using awareness. The time comes, however, when even a positive cycle needs to be terminated using non-attachment.

Impressions of the events of early childhood and the memory of past births in the unconscious mind are the most important factors that determine the pattern of reactions in an individual mind. We have already discussed how chitta, the memory bank, influences buddhi, the decision-making entity. When a person spends the first seven formative years of life in a secure, loving and happy environment, that person's mind is more likely to be conditioned to react in an optimistic, creative and cheerful way. Such a person is more likely to develop healthy personality traits and less likely to succumb to diseases easily. All adults, and especially parents and teachers, should always bear this in mind in their relationships with children.

29

Body-mind connection

When one thinks or feels or experiences something in the mind, a corresponding electrical and chemical (*electrochemical*) change occurs in the brain. The different areas of the brain are closely interconnected. The area named the hypothalamus is important: it receives information from the brain and is a connecting bridge between the somatic (voluntary) nervous system, the autonomic nervous system and the endocrine system. The somatic nervous system controls voluntary activities (such as moving the arm to pick up a pen), the autonomic nervous system has immediate control over involuntary activities of the internal organs (such as digestion and heart rate) and the endocrine system has a long term influence over these involuntary activities. In simple terms, the electrochemical change that occurs in the brain when one thinks or feels or experiences something mentally is transmitted to the hypothalamus and then percolates through the endocrine and nervous systems to the rest of the body. Thus the state of mind can affect, through the hypothalamus, the function of the whole body. The cells of the immune system are also sensitive to changes in the endocrine and autonomic nervous systems (discussed in chapter 2).

Fig. 3.3: Influence of the Mind on the Body

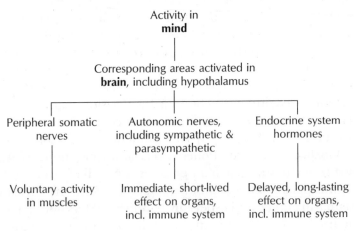

30

The thought patterns, moods and attitudes that a mind harbours influence the internal environment of the body at the physical level. A happy, contented, confident and peaceful mind generally leads to a strong immune system which is possibly more likely to be able to nip the cancer in the bud. Such an immune system may identify the attack and kill the abnormal cancerous cell the moment it comes into existence. It is more likely to allow all the body organs to function freely and optimally in a disease-free environment. By contrast, it is postulated that a mind that is under the influence of stress, worry, frustration, insecurity, discontent, agitation, guilt, jealousy, boredom and hopelessness is more likely to result in a weak immune system. Various body organs may start malfunctioning and the immune system may be too weak to fight against the cancer or other disease. The negative state of mind activates and brings to the surface past negative impressions and experiences. It is more likely to lead to addictions to harmful substances, such as tobacco. This leads to further suffering and entry into a vicious circle until a major disease, such as cancer, may develop.

Researchers have found receptors of catecholamines, prostaglandins, growth hormones, thyroid hormones, sex hormones, serotonin and endorphins on the surface of white blood cells, suggesting the influence of the mind and emotions on the body's immunity by interactions between the nervous, endocrine and immune systems.

THEORY OF KARMA

The theory of karma says that every action, good or bad, bears the appropriate fruit or result either immediately or in the future, including in future lives. When the fruit of a previous action ripens (is activated), its effect is irreversible. One has to undergo it – no force in the universe can change its course. It is better, at this time, to accept the situation as an unavoidable one and flow with it as best we can. But when the fruit of a given action is still in a dormant form, it can be

31

strengthened or weakened by an appropriate action. One must utilize this opportunity to the maximum by being conscious of one's actions and interactions. The spiritual principle, 'Be good, Do good,' is preached by all religions and spiritual movements of the world. The theory of karma applies equally to all without any exception. Karma carries on life after life and is the cause of future births. According to the theory of karma, a negative thought pattern hastens the maturation process of the fruits of past ill actions, resulting in a disease.

Some people strongly believe cancer to be a karmic condition. In the absence of all known causative or contributory factors, people with pure and positively inclined minds also develop cancer in their bodies. This applies to small children and saints like Ramakrishna Paramahamsa and Sri Ramana Maharshi. This can only be explained by the karmic theory for the origin of cancer.

Fig. 3.4: Theory of Karma

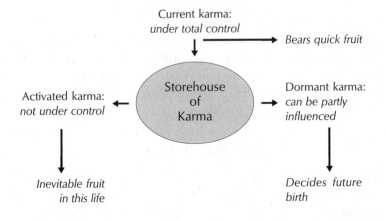

4

A Perspective on the Gunas

Gunas – inherent qualities

Take a little time to look around yourself. Observe human beings, animals and plants as well as non-living things. You will find a pattern amongst their diverse characteristics. For example, they may be energetic and focused, dynamic but scattered, or lethargic. Or they may be peaceful, or disturbed, or inert.

In the Indian tradition it is called the play of *Prakriti*, Mother Nature. Prakriti is made of three qualities, the three *gunas* – sattwa, rajas and tamas, which exist in a state of equilibrium when she is in the dormant state. When the gunas lose their state of equilibrium, prakriti becomes active and creation takes place, evolution starts and the cycle of birth and death begins. When they regain their perfect equilibrium, involution begins, creation dissolves and the cycle of birth and death comes to an end. Thus the gunas are both the cause of creation and also the inherent qualities of all that is created. For example, a stone has inherent qualities of solidity, heaviness and immobility; a river has inherent qualities of fluidity, coolness and transparency, and a deer has agility and tenderness as its inherent qualities.

Each and everything that exists in this universe, therefore, is under the influence of these gunas. The way we think and act is constantly influenced by the gunas. As already discussed in chapter 3, our thoughts, attitudes and actions decide our future desires. As long as we have unfulfilled desires and the fruits of actions that have not been lived through, we continue in the birth-death cycle. The quality of these desires and the fruits of actions that are not yet lived through decide the nature of the next birth. Thus they bind the self, *atman*, to the cycle of life and death by drawing it into the wheel of karma. The *Bhagavad Gita* (14:5) says: "Purity, passion and inertia – these gunas, qualities born of Prakriti, bind fast the indestructible Atman, the Self, to the body."

Types of gunas

These gunas can be identified by their unique characteristics. The first one among them is *sattwa*. It is characterized by luminosity, peace, purity, contentment, balance between opposing forces, positive states, knowledge, righteousness, equanimity, maturity, simplicity and other such qualities. The second guna is *rajas*. It is characterized by passion, activity, dominance, involvement, growth, desire, wrong knowledge, complexity, suffering and other such qualities. The third guna, *tamas,* is characterized by inactivity, dullness, darkness, impurity, decay, negative states, ignorance, delusion and other such qualities.

The *Bhagavad Gita* (14:6–8) describes sattwa as stainless, luminous and healthy and as that which binds the Atman by attachment to happiness and knowledge. Rajas it describes as having the nature of passion, being the source of thirst and attachment, and which binds the atman by attachment to action. Tamas it describes as deluding, born of ignorance and as that which binds the atman fast by heedlessness, indolence and sleep.

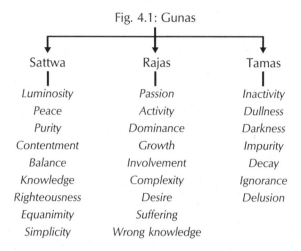

Fig. 4.1: Gunas

Sattwa	Rajas	Tamas
Luminosity	Passion	Inactivity
Peace	Activity	Dullness
Purity	Dominance	Darkness
Contentment	Growth	Impurity
Balance	Involvement	Decay
Knowledge	Complexity	Ignorance
Righteousness	Desire	Delusion
Equanimity	Suffering	
Simplicity	Wrong knowledge	

The gunas always exist in combination. Nothing can be made up of pure sattwa or only rajas or tamas. One of the gunas may dominate while others provide a support on which the predominant one can stand, or they may exist in different permutations and combinations. In general the lower forms of life and non-living things represent tamas guna. As the life form evolves rajas guna appears in increasing amounts. Sattwa guna is found interspersed everywhere in nature and in various life forms.

The dynamics of the gunas are ever-changing. At no two moments can the status of the gunas be the same in a given individual or a situation. Our thoughts and behaviour patterns are constantly under the spell of the play of the gunas. When sattwa predominates we think and act in a given way, but when rajas is dominant we think and behave differently, and when tamas dominates we think and act in yet another way. Our personality type is decided by which guna predominates overall.

However, we need not be a passive puppet dancing to the tune of the gunas. The gunas are changing spontaneously and can also be changed at will. With our conscious will we can change the dominance of a particular guna and bring in the guna of our choice. For example, when a job has a

35

deadline and at midnight we want to ward off sleep, we drink a cup of strong coffee or take a cold shower to change tamas into rajas. When one wants to change a guna to suit the demands of the situation, then an appropriate guna can be brought in by thoughts and actions conducive to that guna. Overall in one's personality tamas should be minimized first by bringing in rajas, and then rajas overcome by enhancing sattwa. The ultimate aim is to go beyond sattwa, that is, not to be interested or attached to the sattwic state, but to remain non-attached and balanced in all the states.

The influence of the gunas on health

According to Ayurveda and yoga, disturbance in the gunas, usually excessive rajas or tamas, leads to ill health. Too much rajas causes diseases such as anxiety, irritable bowel syndrome, high blood pressure, angina and other heart conditions, diabetes and hormonal imbalance, to name just a few. Excess tamas may cause depression, obesity, infections, tumours, degenerative disorders such as arthritis, dementia and other conditions of this nature. *Cancer is a manifestation of accumulated tamas guna.* Sometimes both rajas and tamas are deranged together in different proportions, leading to diseases. Sattwa is a state of balance and good health.

Cancer and tamas guna

Let us consider the effects of tamas in greater detail. According to yoga an individual has five *koshas* or bodies:
1. Annamaya kosha or the physical body
2. Pranamaya kosha or the energy body
3. Manomaya kosha or the mental body
4. Vijnanamaya kosha or the body of wisdom where knowledge is kept in coded form
5. Anandamaya kosha or the body of bliss.
(For more details on the koshas refer to chapter 5.)

Tamas can accumulate at one or more levels of the koshas. In *annamaya kosha*, the physical body, tamas accumulates due to conditions such as poor functioning of the digestive system, intake of unhealthy substances in food, water or air or via the skin, infection with viruses or bacteria, unhealthy lifestyle (for example, inadequate rest or unbalanced activities) and ageing.

In *pranamaya kosha*, the energy body, accumulation of tamas is due to over-exhaustion, exposure to bad weather (e.g. in cold, damp weather stiffness and minor body ache may be experienced), lack of adequate physical activity, lack of interest and enthusiasm.

In *manomaya kosha*, the mental body, tamas can overpower the conscious and subconscious mind, due to wrong knowledge, non-righteous thoughts and behaviour, and related limiting states of mind such as anger, greed, attachment, arrogance, jealousy, animosity, guilt and low self-esteem.

Tamas also influences the deeper layers of the mind or the unconscious mind, known as *vijnanamaya kosha*, the wisdom body. Memories of great impact and impressions of the past, including previous births and impressions of the collective unconscious of the race, are stored in and made available from this level of our being. *Karmaphala*, the consequences or rewards, positive or otherwise, of our behaviour and thoughts, are also stored here. As vijnanamaya kosha is a storehouse, its quality depends upon what goes in. The tamasic way of living and the tamasic interpretation of life-experiences discolour vijnanamaya kosha in a tamasic way. For instance, the company of an addict will keep pulling a young person into negatively charged circumstances; a seed of jealousy will impair a person's thinking and behaviour patterns and lead to negative interpersonal relationships; and a fault-finding nature or pessimism drastically changes the interpretation and experience of life-situations. When the information going to vijnanamaya kosha is repetitive or creates a deep impact, it may be transferred to the consciousness and be lived out through destiny life after life.

The final and subtlest level of our existence is *anandamaya kosha*, the bliss body. We exist there in a blissful state in the form of pure consciousness. This is the state of pure sattwa. In this kosha we are very close to our soul, self or atman.

To summarize, cancer can be considered a result of the accumulation of tamas in one or more koshas.

- Different carcinogens, as described in chapter 3 under the heading of environmental, lifestyle and biological factors, accumulate in the form of various toxins in annamaya kosha, the physical body, over a period of years, eventually potentially leading to cancer.
- When the energy system of the body is not optimal, one or more of the body's functions suffer. When an excess of tamas in pranamaya kosha is long-standing, the body's defence mechanism may become weak, and may fail to identify or destroy abnormal cells in the initial stage.
- Similarly, negative states of mind, tamas in manomaya kosha, can also deplete the immune system, potentially allowing the seeds of cancer to gain the upper hand. This aspect has been discussed in chapter 3.
- Tamas in vijnanamaya kosha is due to negative past karmas. Tamas in this kosha promotes the activation of negative karmas. Cancer may be a manifestation of this. Refer to the discussion of the theory of karma in chapter 3.

2: Understanding the Self

5

Who is the Self?

"We are a soul with a body, not a body with a soul."

Who am I?

If the question 'Who are you?' is asked, instantaneously we will become aware of our body and the answer that emerges will be 'my (this body's) name is so and so'. A longer answer may include family background, the place we come from, our qualifications, the job we are involved in, and so on. These answers come from our identification with the body and the different roles that this body plays.

If we think seriously about the question 'Who am I?' many answers will come forth in a sequence. According to the philosophy of Samkhya, from which the philosophy of yoga originates, all living beings are born with *ahamkara*, awareness of self-identity, to varying degrees. We are also trained by society from our very early days that 'I am this body with this name'. So, that is our first answer to the question, 'Who are you?' In the next few answers we are likely to describe the different roles we play at home, at work and in society. Next we start assigning different qualities to ourselves. What type of a person we are, what our strengths and weaknesses are, what we like and dislike, what our habits and attitudes are, what our instincts are and in which direction they take us, what our aims, ambitions and absolute needs are and so on. But rarely is a person able to go beyond these

41

answers. With yoga we can learn about all these aspects of ourselves in greater detail and more clearly, plus something more – our essential, inner nature, the atman.

The five koshas

The yogic concept of human existence is that our consciousness, termed *atman,* is eternal, non-changeable and all-knowing. When this atman takes birth on this planet, it is covered by five sheaths. The gross sheath of the physical body is called *annamaya kosha. Anna* means food and *kosha* is sheath. It is the container in which the atman resides. Next is the sheath of energy, *pranamaya kosha. Prana* is energy. It nourishes all the other sheaths and is the driving energy behind them. Nothing can function in its absence. Next is the mind, *manomaya kosha.* It receives information, understands and makes decisions. It is the manager of the system. The next sheath, which is subtler still, is the wisdom sheath, *vijnanamaya kosha.* It is the storehouse of knowledge acquired in the past, including past lives. It is also the storehouse of past karmas. It is the director of the system. The last and most subtle sheath, *anandamaya kosha,* reflects our original untainted character of bliss and purity. Wrapped inside all the five coverings is our true 'self' or atman. It watches passively, like a witness, all that goes on outside and inside the being, without being affected.

This concept of atman and the five koshas will become clearer with an example. The body is a chariot driven by horses, which are the energy or prana. The driver of the chariot, the mind, is holding a definite plan of the route in his hand, the vijnanamaya kosha. This guides him to his destination. The master of the chariot, the atman, is sitting behind the driver clad in his beautiful robe, the anandamaya kosha. He is a silent spectator throughout the journey of life.

Learning to know ourselves

We definitely know our annamaya kosha, the physical body, to a large extent, but not fully. We are not so aware of our internal organs, their functioning and their wellbeing. The main principle of yoga practices is 'awareness'. When we sharpen our awareness during different yogic practices, we start learning much more about our body and the effects of its interactions with the environment. We learn to listen to our bodies and choose appropriate actions. While practising asanas, our whole attention is guided to the body part that is moving and the different sensations that arise in the body. Similarly, while practising pranayama, our awareness is focused on the process of breathing and its effect on the body and mind. In meditation we totally introvert our awareness. We become intently aware of the states of the different areas of the body in the beginning and at the end of the practice. While eating, we become aware of the effects of the food on us. This training in awareness even alerts us to the effects of the environment on us. A yoga practitioner's capacity to know his body and its welfare multiplies in many ways.

We know that we are not only this body. The body is only a collection of matter. There is a driving force, an energy that moves our body, making it function. That energy is prana. We usually perceive it as feeling of tiredness versus liveliness, heat versus cold, lightness versus heaviness, alertness versus dullness or drowsiness, and in the form of movement, different moods and the force behind an emotion. We come to know more about our pranamaya kosha through yoga. The cleansing practices called *shatkarma*, the practices of asana, pranayama and pratyahara (relaxation and internalization of awareness) and the principle of awareness are particularly helpful. During asana, as we move our body we consciously bring about a shift in the energy pattern. We feel pain, stiffness and heaviness being replaced by flexibility, lightness and warmth. Our mood changes and we become more alert and interested in our environment. In pranayama as we start breathing deeply, quietly and in a controlled way, we recognize our energy levels changing. We feel more energetic, lighter, clear-headed, warm and peaceful, and the mind becomes steady. In pratyahara and dharana practices the mind is put to a certain task, towing the energy along.

The energy sensations are easily perceived by a one-pointed, concentrated mind. Thus the energy or pranic levels are detected and manipulated to our advantage by yogic practices.

While doing yogic practices, we are constantly asked to observe their effects on the mind and to observe what the mind is doing at that moment. We watch our thoughts coming, staying for a while and disappearing. We watch our moods and emotions. We observe the memory flashes. We learn a lot about the characteristics and functioning of the mind as we constantly keep observing it. Also, as we are attempting pratyahara and dharana (concentration) practices, the mind reveals itself in a more naked form.

Non-practitioners of yoga can also know about their body, energy system and mind reasonably well if they decide to put their mind to it. But beyond this it will be difficult. A yoga practitioner easily learns about his annamaya, pranamaya and manomaya koshas. One also has glimpses of oneself beyond these koshas and into vijnanamaya and anandamaya koshas. Visions, sparks of intuition, a guiding voice or a strong conviction seemingly coming from nowhere, but still very strongly true, are experienced. There are glimpses of the treasure of knowledge that one does not consciously know one possesses, knowledge that one has never actually learnt in this life. This is vijnanamaya kosha, the wisdom sheath. Young children have access to this inner wisdom. Yoga also gives immense feelings of pleasure, peace, harmony and fulfilment. This is anandamaya kosha.

Beyond the five koshas – the atman

Anandamaya kosha, however, is not the end. Beyond that lies our true and essential self, the atman. Vedic and other eastern philosophies believe that a living being is pure consciousness, atman, enveloped by matter and energy. The atman is eternal, subject to no changes and all-knowing. Its outer three sheaths are subject to change, decay and destruction. At the end of a life, the annamaya, pranamaya and manomaya koshas disintegrate and the atman with its two inner subtle sheaths, vijnanamaya and anandamaya koshas, continues in the cycle of birth and death. In death, only the body, prana and mind die; the wisdom body, bliss body and individual consciousness, atman, continue to live on life after life. The *Bhagavad Gita* clearly describes this phenomenon.

It (the soul) is never born nor does it ever die; after having been it again ceases not to be. It is without birth, eternal, changeless and ancient. It does not get destroyed when the body is destroyed. (2:20)

Just as in this body the embodied (soul) passes into childhood, youth and old age, so also does it pass into another body. (2:13)

As a person discards an old garment and puts on a new one, similarly the occupant of the body (the soul) discards the old incapable body and enters a new one. (2:22)

Everything that is born must perish one day and after destruction it is sure to get a new life. Therefore it is not worth grieving over something that is inevitable. (2:27)

The individual self is part of the all-pervading Cosmic Self, in the same way that a pot immersed in an ocean has water inside itself (atman) and is also surrounded by water (*Paramatman*, the Cosmic Self). When the atman realizes its true source, the cosmic consciousness or Paramatman or the higher Self, it merges with it (the pot is not necessary, the water inside and outside merge with each other) and then there is no more birth and death for that atman. This self can be contacted and known during meditation. As the internalized awareness travels into deeper levels of one's own existence during meditation, the atman reveals itself. The *Katha Upanishad* describes it as follows.

The Atman that is subtler than the subtlest, and greater than the greatest, is seated in the cavity of the heart in each living being. One who is free from willing and wishing, with the mind and senses composed, beholds the majesty of the Self and becomes free from sorrow.   (2:20)

This Atman cannot be attained by study of the Vedas, nor through intellect, nor by much hearing. It is attained by one who chooses (prays to) this (Atman) alone. To him this Atman reveals its true nature.   (2:23)

His form is not to be seen. No one beholds Him with the eyes. By controlling the mind, by the intellect and incessant meditation He is revealed. Those who know this (Brahman) become immortal.   (6:9)

Need to connect with the self in cancer

It is the most essential and pressing need of every being to connect to the self, whether they recognize and acknowledge this or not. When we start connecting to our self, the understanding of our body, energy system, mind and its functioning improves. We therefore start to handle and utilize these faculties better, and learn to tap an unlimited inner source of strength and wisdom. One's interactions with other people and the environment become pleasant and growth-promoting. Life starts flowing smoothly. Feelings of contentment, harmony and causeless joy generally prevail.

For people with cancer this need to connect with the self is even stronger. This is because in addition to all of the above:

1. They need to activate this inner power of healing
2. They need this internal support to face the crisis
3. They need to summon their willpower and all their strength to fight and overpower cancer and the associated difficulties
4. Finally, but very importantly, they need the wisdom to know how much to fight, and when to accept gracefully and make the most of a situation that has become irreversible. The need at this stage feels very urgent because the person has become very aware of the vulnerability of life.

YOGA PRACTICES FOR CONNECTING
WITH THE SELF

The meaning of the word *yoga* is connecting with the self. Yoga comes from the Sanskrit verb *yuj*, meaning 'to unite'. Yoga means union, union of oneself with one's higher Self. *Yoga vidya*, the science of yoga, deals with the process of uniting and the various means used for the purpose. The essential nature of the self is *sat*, eternal existence, *chit*, pure consciousness, and *ananda*, bliss. All three gunas are in equilibrium, a state closely mimicked by the predominance of sattwa. The process of uniting involves minimizing tamas and rajas, allowing sattwa to fill up the whole being.

Awareness of the present in time and space is the most important key for connecting to the self. This training of being mindful of everything within and around us allows us to understand our body and mind in relation to the environment. We watch how our body responds to different experiences. We observe our thoughts, their origins (our desires, *iccha*) and how they influence our behaviour (action, *karma*). We also observe the effects of various states of mind on the physiology of the body. Awareness initiates the process of learning about and improving oneself.

Any balanced program of yoga practices is helpful in establishing this connection. We recommend here some selected practices for ready reference. The practices are described at the practice section at the end of this chapter with their general precautions as well as those for cancer patients. It is essential that the practices be selected and learnt under the guidance of a qualified yoga teacher as each individual's needs and capacities are different. It is definitely inadvisable to read a book and then experiment on the self or others.

The practices can be grouped under the following headings:
• Asana
• Breath awareness

47

- Pranayama
- Yoga nidra
- Pratyahara and dharana meditations
- Bhakti yoga
- Mantra japa.

Asana

One begins by connecting with the body, as it is the most easily approachable kosha, by practising some very simple asanas such as:
- Pawanmuktasana part 1 group
- Tadasana (palm tree pose)
- Tiryaka tadasana (swaying palm tree pose)
- Kati chakrasana (waist rotating pose)
- Marjari-asana (cat stretch pose)
- Makarasana (crocodile pose)/saral bhujangasana (easy cobra pose).

The awareness should be directed inside the body where the movements are taking place. These asanas are very gentle, so almost everyone is able to do them. They do not create any harmful effects. Practise them as much as you can comfortably. The quality of awareness is more important than the number of rounds or achieving perfection. *Asana Pranayama Mudra Bandha,* a Yoga Publications Trust publication, is recommended for further reading.

As one becomes adept at the physical aspect of the practice, one starts to synchronize the breath with the physical movement according to the guidance of a teacher. This changes the quality of awareness into a meditative one. The focus of awareness is on the physical body, its internal areas and the mind. The interactions between sensory input from the external environment and one's own being are witnessed during the practice through continual awareness of how the body, the internal organs, the thoughts and feelings respond to different external inputs. In this way we learn about the physical body, prana and the state of mind.

Breath awareness

Breathing naturally and spontaneously, we simply observe each ingoing and outgoing breath closely. Without altering the pattern of breathing, we watch how the breath enters the body, where it goes, how deep or shallow it is, how fast or slowly it flows, how it reverses its path and leaves the body, what sensations it creates as it flows in and out, what happens to the energy level in the body as the breath flows in and out and what goes on inside the mind simultaneously as awareness of the breath continues.

This practice directs the normally extroverted mind to turn inward and become attentive to what is happening inside. It is a very easy and simple practice and at the same time very profound. It makes the mind quiet and brings it to a centre. Mental turmoil stops or one is able to observe it with a neutral attitude and find a way out. If the mind is already calm and balanced it sets it on its inner journey towards the higher self. Breath awareness is an effective tool with a wide range of applications, from release of normal day-to-day stress and management of various disease states to the highest spiritual quest. It can be practised by every age group, all levels of intellect, anywhere, in all physical states and in most emotional states.

Pranayama

After the initial preparation of the body and mind with these basic asanas and breath awareness, the pre-pranayama and pranayama practices are learnt, that is, learning to control the length and depth of the breath. The following are recommended:
• Abdominal breathing
• Thoracic breathing
• Yogic breathing
• Observing the duration of inhalation and exhalation
• Manipulating the length of inhalation and exhalation to a desired ratio
• Nadi shodhana pranayama
• Ujjayi pranayama.

The breath is a vehicle of prana. We connect to the universal energy, or cosmic prana, or prakriti, through our breath. We constantly derive energy from and send out our energy to the cosmos through the breath. All living beings link with each other and with the cosmos through their breath and thoughts. The breath also serves as a bridge between the body and mind. The state of the mind and body can be manipulated by manipulating the breath. By modifying the pattern of breathing we can modify the physical, pranic and mental states. Various pranayama practices offer this possibility. We can understand and adjust our pranamaya and manomaya koshas with pranayama practices.

Precaution: Pranayama should only be practised according to the capacity of the individual. Never use force or put the lungs under undue strain. Practise only under the guidance of a qualified teacher. People with high blood pressure or any heart problem should not practise inner or outer *kumbhaka*, breath retention, except under expert guidance. (*Asana Pranayama Mudra Bandha*, a Yoga Publications Trust publication, is recommended for further reading.)

Yoga nidra

Yoga nidra is a guided practice of relaxation and *pratyahara* (withdrawing the mind from external sense objects and directing it inward). It was first devised by Swami Satyananda Saraswati based on knowledge of the ancient tantric texts. In this progressive relaxation practice, the relaxation gradually deepens from the muscular level to the mental, emotional and deep psychic levels, enabling the practitioner to enter and explore the deeper layers of the mind one by one. The contents of the mind spontaneously surface. Long forgotten impressions can rise into the conscious realm. This helps us to understand many of our attitudes, habits and reactions in the light of this newfound knowledge.

It is only possible to connect with the self when in a totally relaxed state. If anything is bothering the body or the mind, this connection is not possible unless one learns to transcend that disturbance consciously and then relax at will. The practice of yoga nidra provides this training and also the opportunity for this practice and experience. (*Yoga Nidra*, a Yoga Publications Trust publication, is recommended for further reading.)

Pratyahara and dharana meditations

In pratyahara practices the mind is withdrawn from external sense objects and directed inwards. Dharana practice is the next stage, where the introverted mind is given a focus to attach itself to. Normally both these stages are practised together in succession. As the mind becomes absorbed in one-pointed awareness on the given focus of concentration, rajas decreases and the state of sattwa predominance manifests, leading the practitioner into states of *dhyana*, undisturbed focused awareness. In this state of true meditation, the original, untainted nature of the higher self is revealed and yoga, union, occurs. Pratyahara and dharana practice trains us to connect with the atman, the inner source of life. With this, we start drawing on our inner strength, becoming self reliant. The recommended practices are: antar mouna, ajapa japa, trataka and mantra japa.

In the practice of antar mouna the focus of attention is on the thoughts and in ajapa japa on the breath and sound. In trataka the focus of attention is a visual symbol. It can be a candle flame (*jyoti*) or a personal symbol representing higher consciousness (*ishta deva*). In the practice of mantra meditation, sound is utilized.

Antar mouna: The Sanskrit word *antar* means inner and *mouna* means silence. In this pratyahara practice the coming and going of the thoughts is observed in the passive manner of a witness. This process of just observing brings many forgotten or suppressed issues to the surface, i.e. to the level of conscious recognition. These can then be dealt with and settled in a manner appropriate for that individual. A mental catharsis takes place and then the mind becomes comparatively quiet and at peace with itself. Thoughts also arise during

51

any dharana practice or work demanding concentration. The process of antar mouna should simultaneously continue.

Ajapa japa: *Japa* means repetition of mantra, and *ajapa* means spontaneous repetition without conscious effort. The practice of ajapa japa involves rotation of the consciousness in a psychic passage using mantra and breath, initially consciously. This introverts the mind fairly quickly. It is a combination of pranayama and dharana practice. The benefits are wide ranging, from calming and de-stressing effects to the highest goal of self-realization.

Trataka means to gaze steadily. A still body, still senses (minimum sensory input) and slow rhythmic breath allow the mind to slow down and also become still. A still mind quickly introverts and can start connecting to the self. In trataka one attempts to still the mind through stilling the most active, wandering sense organ, the eye. This practice also encourages inner wisdom to unfold in the form of symbols and visions. Trataka is also used in bhakti yoga.

The practice of mantra japa is dealt with below. (*Dharana Darshan, Meditations from the Tantras, Sure Ways to Self-Realization* and *Yoga and Kriya*, published by Yoga Publications Trust, are recommended for further reading.)

Precaution: In the early stages a practitioner needs to be guided by a teacher. Later, when the practice is understood, an audio recording, if applicable, can be used. Once the practice is known and the practitioner feels confident, it can be done independently. Pratyahara and dharana practices may not work well with depressed or introverted people. It is generally advised that people with a history of mental disorders should refrain from dharana practices except under expert guidance.

Bhakti yoga

One can also take up the path of bhakti yoga. Bhakti is faith and pure love for a higher reality of life, the higher cosmic force, or God. In bhakti yoga one tries to build a relationship with God. It can take the form of a relationship between parent and child, two lovers, two friends, master and servant or any other type that feels right and natural. The feeling should be effortless, not forced. Such a relationship offers unfailing support. Bhakti is not religion; it is a science of inner transformation. It changes the thinking patterns and basic tendencies, and purifies and stabilizes the emotions effectively by channelling them to a higher reality. In trying to know the object of devotion deeply, one realizes that the devotee and the beloved are one, not two different entities. The knowledge that the beloved resides in one's own heart dawns and knowledge of the inner self is revealed.

Singing in praise of God, hearing stories of His deeds, chanting His name, worshipping Him, thinking deeply about Him and surrendering to Him are the main practices of bhakti yoga. They are discussed at length in the practice section at the end of this chapter and in chapter 7. (*Upasana: In the Presence of the Divine* and *Samarpan: Living the Divine Connection,* published by Yoga Publications Trust, are recommended for further reading.)

Mantra japa

Mantra japa is a pratyahara and dharana practice in the raja yoga tradition and also a very important practice of bhakti yoga. The word *japa* means to rotate, and *japa yoga* means union with the highest existence through mantra repetition or rotation of consciousness. In mantra japa the selected mantra, usually of a few syllables, is repeated over and over, either verbally, whispering or mentally, using a *mala*, a string of 108 beads. In the practice of *likhit japa*, the mantra is written down. Faith and awareness are helpful for the practice. For many practioners, lighting a *deepak* or candle, incense, offering flowers and other similar simple actions or rituals help make the external atmosphere conducive to the practice, while simultaneously touching the heart of the practitioner who is making a humble offering and invoking purity.

The repetitive sound vibrations of mantra produce a vibratory force that works subtly on the psyche and awakens it. Mantra becomes the bridge that links the conscious mental faculty with the deeper psyche and the inner self. Mantra japa is an ancient and universal practice followed by most religions and cultures. It is a common spiritual practice in Hinduism, Christianity, Sufism and Buddhism, to name just a few of the major faiths.

Fig. 5.1: Practices for Connecting to the Self

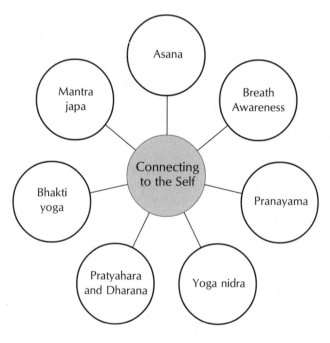

ASANA

General notes for the practitioner

Breathing: Always breathe through the nose unless specific instructions are given to the contrary. Coordinate the breath with the asana practice.

Awareness: This is as essential to the practice of asana as it is to all yoga practices. The purpose of asana practice is to influence, integrate and harmonize all levels of being: physical, pranic, mental, emotional, psychic and spiritual. Awareness in this context may be understood as consciously noting sensations in the body, the physical movement, the posture itself, breath control and synchronization and, most importantly, witnessing any thoughts or feelings that may arise during the practice. This awareness is essential in order to receive optimum benefits from the practices.

Relaxation: Shavasana may be performed at any point during asana practice, especially when feeling physically or mentally tired. It should also be practised on completion of the asana program.

Sequence: After completing the shatkarmas, asanas should be done, followed by pranayamas, then pratyahara and dharana, which lead to meditation.

---

*The practices in this section follow the sequence in which they should be learned and practised.

Time of practice: Asanas may be practised at any time of day except after meals. The best time, however, is the two hours before and including sunrise. The atmosphere is pure and quiet, the stomach and intestines are inactive, the mind has no deep impressions on the conscious level and is relatively empty of thoughts in preparation for the day ahead. In the evening, the two hours around sunset is also a favourable time.

Place of practice: Practice should be done in a room that is naturally well ventilated and where it is calm and quiet. Asanas may also be practised outdoors, but the surroundings should be pleasant, for example, in a beautiful garden with trees and flowers. Do not practise in a strong wind, in the cold, in air that is dirty, smoky or which carries an unpleasant odour. Do not practise in the vicinity of furniture, a fire or anything that can cause injury. Do not practise under an electric fan unless it is extremely hot.

Yoga mat: Use a folded blanket of natural material for the practices to provide insulation between the body and the floor or ground. Do not use a mattress which is spongy or filled with air as it will not give sufficient support to the spine.

Clothes: Wear loose, light and comfortable clothing. Before commencing, remove spectacles, wrist watches and any jewellery.

Bathing: Try to take a shower (cold if possible) before starting. This will greatly improve the effect of the asanas.

Emptying the bowels: The bladder and intestines should preferably be empty.

Empty stomach: The stomach should be empty while doing asanas. For this reason, asanas should not be practised until at least three or four hours after food. This is one reason why early morning practice is recommended as the stomach is sure to be empty.

Diet: There are no special dietary rules for asana practitioners, although it is better to eat natural food and in moderation. Contrary to popular belief, yoga does not say that a vegetarian diet is essential, although in the higher stages of practice it is recommended. At meal times it is advised to half fill the stomach with food, one quarter with water and leave the remaining quarter empty. Eat only to satisfy hunger and not so much that a feeling of heaviness or laziness occurs. Eat to live rather than live to eat. Foods which cause acidity or gas in the digestive system, or which are heavy, oily and spicy, should be avoided, especially when asanas are practised with a spiritual aim.

No straining: Never exert undue force while doing asanas.

Contra-indications: People with cardiac problems or hernia, and those recuperating from operations, should consult a competent yoga teacher or doctor before commencing asanas. Carefully observe the contra-indications given for individual asanas.

Termination of asana: If there is excessive pain in any part of the body, the asana should be stopped immediately and if necessary, medical advice sought. Do not stay in an asana if discomfort is felt.

For cancer patients: Avoid direct compression of the tumour or lesion and strain on any bone with metastasis.

PAWANMUKTASANA PART 1

There are no overall contra-indications for practising this series. An immobile, bed-ridden person can also do these practices. The benefits and contra-indications for individual practices are given with each practice.

General benefits

This series of asanas improves blood circulation in the respective area by enhancing the venous return. Lymphatic drainage is also improved. These asanas are therefore useful in relieving pain, swelling and inflammation and in speeding up healing. They also boost the immune system, are introverting and help sharpen awareness of the internal organs and tissues.

Benefits in specific cancers

- Practices 1–4 should be practised when confined to bed, with limited movement or post-operatively.
- Practices 11–15 are very beneficial in breast cancer post-operatively and when there is pain due to intravenous injections.
- Practice 16 is very beneficial in cancer of the head and neck region post-operatively and after radiotherapy
- The whole series should be practised after chemotherapy and in any debilitating condition.

Awareness

The practices may be performed in two ways:

1. With awareness of the actual physical movement, the interaction between the various components of the body, i.e. bones, joints, ligaments, muscles, etc.; the movement in relation to other parts of the body; with mental counting of each completed round; and with awareness of thoughts arising in the mind. This method of practice induces peace, balance and one-pointedness, which in turn brings about harmony in the physical body.
2. With awareness and integrated breathing. In addition to the awareness of physical movement described above, individual movements are synchronized with the breath. The movements become slower, which in turn slows the brain waves, further enhancing relaxation and awareness. This method of practice has a greater influence at the physical and pranic levels and is especially useful for harmonizing and revitalizing the body and improving the functioning of the internal organs. Breathing should be practised as indicated in the description of each asana. In addition, experienced students may find an increased benefit if ujjayi pranayama is used during these asanas. This effectively stimulates and balances the pranic energy flowing through the nadis.

Periodic rest

After every two or three practices, sit quietly in the base position with the eyes closed and be aware of the natural breath, of the part or parts of the body that have just been moved, and of any thoughts or feelings that come into the mind. After a minute or so continue the practice. This will not only rest the body, but will also develop awareness of the internal energy patterns and the mental and emotional processes. This rest period is almost as important as the asanas themselves and should not be neglected.

If tiredness is experienced at any point during the asana program, rest in shavasana. Shavasana should be performed for three to five minutes at the end of the program.

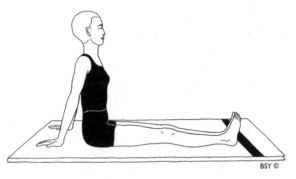

BSY ©

Prarambhik Sthiti (base position)

All the practices of pawanmuktasana part 1 are performed while sitting on the floor in the base position.

Sit with the legs outstretched and the feet together. Place the hands beside and slightly behind the buttocks.

Lean back a little, using the arms to support the back.

Keep the spine straight.

The body should be relaxed, and only those muscles associated with the asana being practised should be used. Full awareness should be given to performance of the asana as per the notes above. For maximum benefit the eyes can remain closed. Do not practise mechanically, be aware throughout the practice.

Practice 1: Padanguli Naman (toe bending)

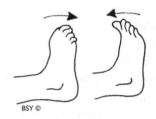

Sit in the base position.

Be aware of the toes. Move only the toes of both feet slowly backward and forward, keeping the feet upright and the ankles relaxed and motionless.

Hold each position for a few seconds.

Repeat 10 times.

Breathing: Inhale as the toes move backward.
Exhale as the toes move forward.

Awareness: On the stretching produced by the movement and the breath.

Practice 2: Goolf Naman (ankle bending)

Remain in the base position.

Slowly move both feet backward and forward, bending them from the ankle joints. Try to stretch the feet forward to touch the floor and then draw them back towards the knees. Hold each position for a few seconds.

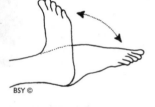

Repeat 10 times.

Breathing: Inhale as the feet move backward.
Exhale as the feet move forward.

Awareness: On the stretch in the foot, ankle, calf and leg, and the breath.

Practice 3: Goolf Chakra (ankle rotation)

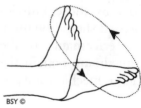

Remain in the base position.
Keep the legs shoulder-width apart and straight.
Keep the heels on the ground throughout the practice.

60

Stage 1: Slowly rotate the right foot clockwise from the ankle 10 times and then repeat 10 times anti-clockwise. Repeat the same procedure with the left foot.

Stage 2: Slowly rotate both feet together in the same direction.

Focus on rotating the feet and not the knees.

Practice 10 times clockwise and then 10 times anti-clockwise.

Stage 3: Keep the feet separated.

Slowly rotate both feet from the ankles together, but in opposite directions.

Do 10 rotations in one direction and then 10 rotations in the opposite direction.

Breathing: Inhale on the upward movement.

Exhale on the downward movement.

Awareness: On the rotation of the ankle and the breath.

Practice 4: Goolf Ghoornan (ankle crank)

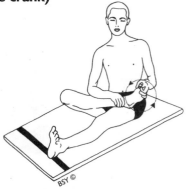

Remain in the base position. Bend the right knee and bring the foot towards the groin. Turn the knee out to the side and if there is no strain, gently place the foot on the left thigh.

Make sure the ankle is far enough over the thigh to be free for rotation.

Hold the right leg a little above the ankle with the right hand.

Hold the toes of the right foot with the left hand.

With the aid of the left hand, slowly rotate the right foot 10 times clockwise, then 10 times anti-clockwise.

Change the leg and repeat with the left foot placed on the right thigh.

Breathing: Inhale on the upward movement.

Exhale on the downward movement.

61

Awareness: On the rotation and the breath.

Benefits of practices 1–4: All the foot and calf asanas help in returning stagnant lymph and venous blood, thus relieving tiredness and cramp, and helping to prevent venous thrombosis, especially in bedridden, post-operative patients.

Practice 5: Janufalak Akarshan (kneecap contraction)

Stay in the base position.

Gently contract the muscle surrounding the right knee, drawing the kneecap back towards the thigh.

Hold the contraction for 3 to 5 seconds, counting mentally.

Release the contraction and let the kneecap return to its normal position.

Practise 10 times. Repeat with the left kneecap 10 times, then with both kneecaps together.

Breathing: Inhale while contracting.

Exhale while relaxing the knee muscles.

Awareness: On the contraction and the breath.

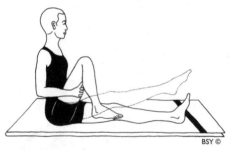

BSY ©

Practice 6: Janu Naman (knee bending)

Stage 1: Stay in the base position. Bend the right knee, bringing the thigh near the chest and clasp the hands under the right thigh.

Straighten the right leg fully.

Keep the hands under the thigh, but straighten the arms. Keep the heel about 10 cms off the floor.

Again bend the right knee so that the thigh comes close to the chest and the heel is near the groin.

Keep the head and spine straight.

This is one round.

Practise 10 rounds with the right leg and then 10 rounds with the left leg.

Stage 2: Bend both knees together, bringing the thighs near the chest and place the feet on the floor in front of the groin.

Hold the backs of the thighs.

Raise the feet slightly from the floor and balance on the buttocks.

Straighten the legs as much as you can without straining. The arms straighten naturally while the hands continue to support the thighs.

Point the toes forward.

The hands and arms should support and maintain the stability of the body. Keep the head and spine upright.

Remain in the position for a few seconds.

Bend the knees and bring the legs back to the starting position, keeping the heels slightly above the floor.

Draw the toes back towards the shins.

This is one round.

Practise 5 to 10 rounds, keeping the heels off the floor throughout the practice.

Breathing: Inhale while straightening the legs.

Exhale while bending the legs.

Awareness: On the knee bend and associated movement and balance, and the breath.

Contra-indications: Stage 2 is a strenuous practice and should not be attempted by people with weak abdominal muscles, back conditions, high blood pressure or heart conditions.

Practice 7: Janu Chakra (knee crank)

Sit in the base position.

Bend the right knee and bring the thigh near the chest.

Place the hands under the right thigh and interlock the fingers or cross the arms holding the elbows.

Raise the right foot from the ground.

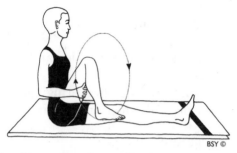

Rotate the lower leg from the knee in a large circular movement; try to straighten the leg at the top of the upward movement.

The upper leg and trunk should be completely still.

Rotate 10 times clockwise and then 10 times anti-clockwise.

Repeat with the left leg.

Breathing: Inhale on the upward movement.

Exhale on the downward movement.

Awareness: On the movement and perfection of the circular rotation, and the breath.

Benefits of practices 5–7: Since the knee joint bears the whole weight of the body and has no strong muscles for support, it is most vulnerable to injuries, sprains and osteoarthritis. All the knee asanas strengthen the quadriceps muscle and the ligaments around the knee joint. These asanas rejuvenate the joint by activating the healing energies.

Practice 8: Ardha Titali Asana (half butterfly)

Sit in the base position.

Bend the right leg and place the right foot comfortably on the left thigh.

Place the right hand on top of the bent right knee.

Hold the toes of the right foot with the left hand.

This is the starting position.

Stage 1: with breath synchronization

While breathing in, gently move the right knee up towards the chest. Breathing out, gently push the knee down and try to touch the knee to the floor.

The trunk should not move.

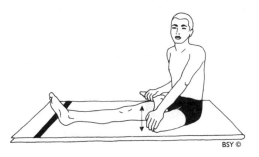

BSY ©

Do not force this movement in any way.

The leg muscles should be passive, the movement being achieved by the exertion of the right arm.

Slowly practise 10 up and down movements.

Awareness: On the movement of the hip joint, relaxation of the inner thigh muscles, and the breath.

Stage 2: without breath synchronization

Remain in the same position with the right leg on the left thigh.

Relax the right leg muscles as much as possible.

Push the right knee down with the right hand and try to touch the knee to the floor.

Do not strain.

Let the knee spring up by itself.

The movement is achieved by using the right arm only.

Practise 30 up and down movements in quick succession.

Breathing should be normal and unrelated to the practice.

Realign the right knee (see the practice note below for the procedure).

Repeat stages 1 and 2 and the realigning procedure with the left leg.

Awareness: On the movement of the knee and hip joints and relaxation of the inner thigh muscles.

Practice note: Gently straighten the leg after completing the practice, then again slowly and carefully bend it once, bringing the heel near the groin, then stretch the leg in front fully.

This procedure will ensure that the knee joint is realigned correctly.

65

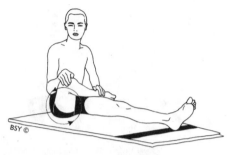

Practice 9: Shroni Chakra (hip rotation)

Sit in the same starting position as for ardha titali asana with the right foot on the left thigh.

Use the right hand to rotate the right knee in a circle and make the circular movement as large as possible.

The index finger may be pointed out and used as a guide to perfection of the circular movement.

Practise 10 rotations clockwise and then 10 rotations anti-clockwise.

Straighten the leg slowly and realign the knees.

Repeat with the left leg.

Breathing: Inhale on the upward movement.

Exhale on the downward movement.

Awareness: On the rotation of the knee, ankle and hip joint, and the breath.

Practice 10: Poorna Titali Asana (full butterfly)

Sit in the base position.

Bend the knees and bring the soles of the feet together, keeping the heels as close to the perineum as possible.

Allow the knees to drop downward and outward as much as possible.

Fully relax the inner thigh muscles.

Stage 1: Clasp the feet with both hands.

Gently move the knees up and then down towards the floor, but do not use any force.

Practise up to 30 up and down movements.

Stage 2: Keep the soles of the feet together.

Place the hands on the knees.

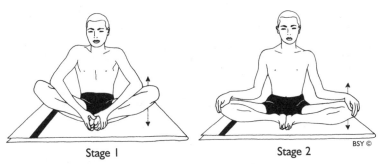

Stage I   Stage 2

Using the hands, gently push the knees down towards the
floor, allowing them to spring up again.

Do not force this movement.

Repeat 10 to 30 times. Straighten the legs, realign the
knees and relax.

Breathing: Normal breathing, unrelated to the practice.

Awareness: On the hip joint, movement and relaxation.

Contra-indications: People with sciatica should avoid this
asana.

Benefits of practices 8–10: They prepare the legs for
meditative asanas. The inner thigh muscles hold a lot of
tension which is relieved by these asanas. They also remove
tiredness due to long hours of standing and walking.

Practice 11: Mushtika Bandhana (hand clenching)

Sit in the base position or a cross-legged
pose.

Hold both arms straight in front of the
body at shoulder level.

Open the hands, palms down, and
stretch the fingers as wide apart as
possible.

Close the fingers to make a tight fist with
the thumbs inside.

The fingers should be slowly wrapped
around the thumbs.

Again open the hands and stretch the fingers.

Repeat 10 times.

67

Breathing: Inhale on opening the hands.
  Exhale on closing the hands.
Awareness: On the stretching sensation and movement, and
  the breath.

Practice 12: Manibandha Naman (wrist bending)

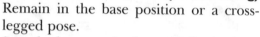

Remain in the base position or a cross-legged pose.

Stretch the arms in front of the body at shoulder level.

Keep the palms open and fingers straight throughout the entire practice.

Bend the hands backward from the wrists as if pressing the palms against a wall with the fingers pointing toward the ceiling.

Bend the hands forward from the wrists so that the fingers point toward the floor.

Keep the elbows straight throughout the practice.

Do not bend the knuckle joints or fingers.

Bend the hands up again for the next round.

Repeat 10 times.

Breathing: Inhale with the backward movement.
  Exhale with the forward movement.
Awareness: On the movement in the wrist joint and stretching
  of the forearm muscles, and the breath.

Practice 13: Manibandha Chakra (wrist joint rotation)

Remain in the base position or a comfortable cross-legged pose, but keep the back straight.

Stage 1: Extend the right arm forward at shoulder level.

Make a loose fist with the right hand, with the thumb inside.

This is the starting position.

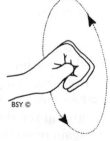

Slowly rotate the fist about the wrist, ensuring that the fist faces downward throughout the rotation.

68

The arms and elbows should remain perfectly straight and still. Make as large a circle as possible.

Practise 10 times clockwise and 10 times anti-clockwise.

Repeat the same with the left fist.

Stage 2: Extend both arms in front of the body with the fists loosely clenched.

Keep the arms straight and at shoulder level.

Rotate the fists together in the same direction.

Practise 10 times in each direction.

Stage 3: Practise as in stage 2 while rotating the fists in opposite directions.

Practise 10 times in each direction.

Benefits of practices 11–13: The hand and wrist asanas are beneficial for the related joints. They also relieve tension caused by prolonged writing, typing and so on.

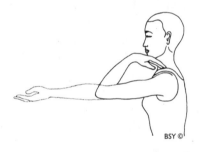

Practice 14: Kehuni Naman (elbow bending)

Stage 1: Remain in the base position or a cross-legged pose. Stretch the arms in front of the body at shoulder level.

The hands should be open with the palms facing up.

Bend the arms at the elbows and touch the fingers to the shoulders. Keep the upper arms parallel to the floor.

Straighten the arms again.

This is one round.

Repeat 10 times.

Stage 2: Extend the arms sideways at shoulder level, hands open and palms facing the ceiling.

Bend the arms at the elbows and touch the fingers to the shoulders. Keep the upper arms parallel to the floor.

Again straighten the arms sideways.

Repeat 10 times.

Breathing: Inhale while straightening the arms.

Exhale while bending the arms.

Awareness: On the movement of the elbow joint and arm muscles, and the breath.

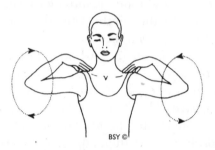

Practice 15: Skandha Chakra (shoulder socket rotation)

Stage 1: Remain in the base position or a cross-legged pose.

Place the fingers of the right hand on the right shoulder.

Keep the left hand on the left knee and the back straight.

Rotate the right elbow in a large circle.

Practise 10 times clockwise and 10 times anti-clockwise.

Repeat with the left elbow.

Make sure that the head, trunk and spine remain straight and still.

Stage 2: Place the fingers of the left hand on the left shoulder and the fingers of the right hand on the right shoulder.

Fully rotate both elbows at the same time in a large circle. Try to touch the elbows in front of the chest on the forward movement and touch the ears while moving up. Stretch the arms back in the backward movement and touch the sides of the trunk while coming down.

Practise slowly 10 times in one direction and then 10 times in the other direction.

Breathing: Inhale on the upper half of the circular movement.

Exhale on the lower half of the circular movement.

Awareness: On the stretching sensation around the shoulder joint and the breath.

Benefits: The shoulder asanas relieve the strain of driving and office work, and are also helpful in cervical spondylitis and frozen shoulder. They maintain the shape of the shoulders and chest. They release stored tension in the neck and shoulder region.

Practice 16: Greeva Sanchalana (neck movements)

Stage 1: Sit in a cross-legged pose with the hands resting on the knees in jnana or chin mudra. Close the eyes. Slowly move the head forward and try to touch the chin to the chest. Move the head as far back as is comfortable. Do not strain. Feel the stretch of the muscles in the front and back of the neck, and the loosening of the vertebrae in the neck. Practise 10 times.

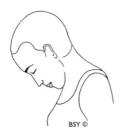

Breathing: Inhale on the backward movement. Exhale on the forward movement.

Stage 2: Remain in the same position, keeping the eyes closed. Face directly forward. Relax the shoulders. Slowly move the head to the right, bringing the right ear close to the right shoulder without raising the shoulders.

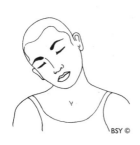

Move the head to the left side and bring the left ear close to the left shoulder. Do not strain; touching the shoulder is not necessary. This is one round. Practise 10 rounds.

Breathing: Inhale on the upward movement. Exhale on the downward movement.

Awareness: On the stretching sensation of the muscles in the sides of the neck, and the breath.

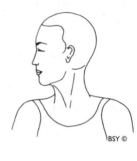

Stage 3: Remain in the same sitting position.

Keep the head upright and the eyes closed.

Gently turn the head to the right so that the chin is in line with the right shoulder.

Feel the release of tension in the neck muscles and the loosening of the neck joints.

Slowly turn the head to the left as far as is comfortable.
Do not strain.

Practise 10 times on each side.

Breathing: Inhale while turning to the front.

Exhale while turning to the side.

Stage 4: Remain in the same position with the eyes closed.

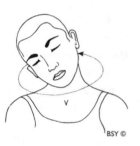

Slowly rotate the head downward, to the right, backward and then to the left side in a relaxed, smooth, rhythmic, circular movement.

Feel the shifting stretch around the neck and the loosening up of the joints and muscles of the neck.

Practise 10 times clockwise and then 10 times anti-clockwise.

Do not strain.

If dizziness occurs, open the eyes and discontinue the practice for that day.

After the practice, keep the neck straight and the eyes closed. Be aware of the sensations in the head and neck.

Breathing: Inhale as the chin moves up.

Exhale as the chin moves down.

Awareness: On the movement and the breath.

Contra-indications: These four neck movements should not be performed by elderly people and those suffering from low blood pressure, high blood pressure, vertigo or giddiness and severe cervical spondylitis. Expert advice should be sought for any of these problems. Cervical disc patients should strictly avoid forward bending of the neck.

Benefits: The muscles of the neck and shoulders accumulate tension, especially after prolonged work at a desk. These asanas release tension, heaviness and stiffness in the head, neck and shoulder region. They massage the major blood vessels supplying the head and neck region and lubricate the joints of the cervical vertebrae.

OTHER ASANAS

Tadasana (palm tree pose)

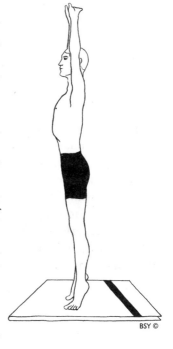

Stand with the feet together or about 10 cm apart, and the arms by the sides.

Steady the body and distribute the weight equally on both feet.

Raise the arms over the head.

Interlock the fingers and turn the palms upward.

Place the hands on top of the head.

Fix the eyes at a point on the wall slightly above the level of the head.

The eyes should remain fixed on this point throughout the practice.

Inhale and stretch the arms, shoulders and chest upward. Raise the heels, coming up onto the toes.

Stretch the whole body from top to bottom, without losing balance or moving the feet.

Hold the breath and the position for a few seconds.

BSY ©

At first it may be difficult to maintain balance, but with practice it becomes easier.

Lower the heels while breathing out and bring the hands to the top of the head.

This is one round.

Relax for a few seconds before performing the next round. Practise 10 rounds.

Breathing: Inhale while raising the arms, retain or breathe normally in the stretch, and exhale while lowering the arms.

Awareness: Physical – on the stretch of the whole body from top to bottom, on maintaining balance and on the breath. Spiritual – initially on mooladhara chakra to provide stability. Once balance is achieved, change to ajna chakra.

Benefits: This asana develops physical and mental balance. The entire spine is stretched and loosened, helping to clear up congestion of the spinal nerves at the points where they emerge from the spinal column. It helps relieve tiredness of body. When done after drinking 2-3 glasses of plain water and followed by tiryaka tadasana and kati chakrasana, it stimulates the digestive system and helps to remove constipation.

Precaution: People with difficulty in maintaining balance or vertigo should practise this asana with due care.

Variation: Tadasana may also be performed while gazing up at the interlocked fingers. It will be slightly more difficult to maintain balance in the final position.

Practice note: Those practitioners who have mastered tadasana with the eyes open may try it with the eyes closed. Tadasana, tiryaka tadasana and kati chakrasana is a popular asana sequence.

Tiryaka Tadasana (swaying palm tree pose)

Stand with the feet more than shoulder width apart.

Fix the gaze on a point directly in front.

Interlock the fingers and turn the palms outward.

Raise the arms over the head, stretching upwards.

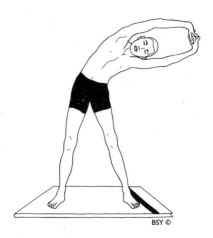

Bend to the right side from the waist.

Do not bend forward or backward or twist the trunk.

Hold the position for a few seconds, then slowly come back to the upright position.

Repeat on the left side. This completes one round.

Practise 10 rounds.

To end the practice, return to the upright position, release the hands, bringing the arms down to the sides.

Breathing: Inhale raising the arms, exhale while bending to the side, inhale to centre. Exhale while releasing the posture.

Awareness: Physical – on keeping the balance and the stretch along the side of the body. On keeping the body and head facing forward while bending to the sides without twisting. On the breath synchronized with the movement.

Spiritual – on mooladhara or manipura chakra.

Benefits: As for tadasana, but it especially massages, loosens and exercises the sides of the waist. It balances the right and left groups of postural muscles.

Precaution: People with difficulty in maintaining balance or vertigo should practise this asana with due care.

Variation: Balance on the toes in this practice.

Practice note: Tadasana, tiryaka tadasana and kati chakrasana is a popular asana sequence.

Kati Chakrasana (waist rotating pose)

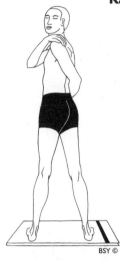

Stand with the feet about shoulder width apart and the arms by the sides.

Raise the arms by the side to shoulder level, then twist the body to the right.

Bring the left hand to the right shoulder and wrap the right arm around the back, bringing the right hand around the left side of the waist. Look over the right shoulder as far as is comfortable.

Keep the back of the neck straight and imagine the top of the spine is the fixed point around which the head turns.

Hold for two seconds, accentuate the twist, gently stretching the abdomen.

Return to the starting position.

Repeat on the other side to complete one round.

Keep the feet firmly on the ground while twisting.

Relax the arms and back as much as possible throughout the practice. Do not strain. The movement should be relaxed and spontaneous.

Perform the rotation smoothly, without jerking or stiffness.

Practise 5 to 10 rounds.

Breathing: Inhale raising the arms.

Exhale twisting to the side.

Inhale returning to the centre.

Exhale while releasing the posture.

Awareness: On the stretch of the abdomen and spinal muscles, and on the breathing synchronized with the movement.

Benefits: This asana tones the neck, shoulders, waist, back and hips. It is useful for correcting back stiffness and postural problems. The relaxation and twisting movement induces a feeling of lightness and may be used to relieve physical and mental tension at any time during the day.

Precaution: People with difficulty in maintaining balance, or vertigo, or knee problems should practise this asana carefully.

Practice note: Tadasana, tiryaka tadasana and kati chakrasana is a popular asana sequence. People with knee problems should make sure that they rotate the body from the waist upwards so that the knees remain pointing forward.

Vajrasana (thunderbolt pose)

Kneel on the floor with the knees close together.

Bring the big toes together and separate the heels.

Lower the buttocks onto the inside surface of the feet with the heels touching the sides of the hips.

Place the hands on the knees, palms down.

The back and head should be straight but not tense.

BSY ©

Avoid excessive backward arching of the spine.

Close the eyes, relax the arms and the whole body.

Breathe normally and fix the attention on the flow of air passing in and out of the nostrils.

Duration: For extended periods of time if performed for spiritual aims. A few minutes daily is sufficient to loosen up the legs. If any strain is experienced, stop the asana. Practise vajrasana directly after meals, for at least 5 minutes to enhance the digestive function. In cases of acute digestive disorder, sit in vajrasana and practise abdominal breathing for 100 breaths before and after food. Do not strain.

Awareness: Physical – on the sensations in the legs, buttocks and spine. When comfortable in the asana become aware of the normal breathing process. This will bring tranquillity to the mind if practised with the eyes closed.

Spiritual – on manipura chakra.

Contra-indications: People with knee problems should not perform this asana.

Benefits: Vajrasana alters the flow of blood and nervous impulses in the pelvic region and strengthens the pelvic muscles. It alleviates menstrual disorders. It increases the efficiency of the entire digestive system.

Vajrasana is a very important meditation posture because the body becomes upright and straight with no effort. It is the best meditation asana for people suffering from sciatica. It stimulates the vajra nadi, activates prana in sushumna and redirects sexual energy for spiritual purposes.

For cancer patients: Vajrasana is especially recommended in cancer of the pelvic organs (cervix, uterus, ovary, urinary, bladder, prostate, rectum, colon etc.), cancer of the testes and cancer of the digestive system (oesophagus, stomach, duodenum, small and large intestines, rectum and anal canal, liver, gall bladder and pancreas).

Practice note: If there is pain in the thighs, the knees may be separated slightly while maintaining the posture.

Beginners may find that their ankles ache after a short time in vajrasana. To remedy this, release the posture, sit with the legs stretched forward and shake the feet vigorously one after the other until the stiffness disappears. Then resume the posture.

Marjari-asana (cat stretch pose)

Sit in vajrasana.

Raise the buttocks and stand on the knees.

Lean forward and place the hands flat on the floor beneath the shoulders with the fingers facing forward.

The hands should be in line with the knees; the arms and thighs should be perpendicular to the floor.

The knees may be slightly separated so that they are well aligned under the hips.

This is the starting position.

Inhale while raising the head and depressing the spine so that the back becomes concave.

Expand the abdomen fully and fill the lungs with the maximum amount of air. Hold the breath for 3 seconds.

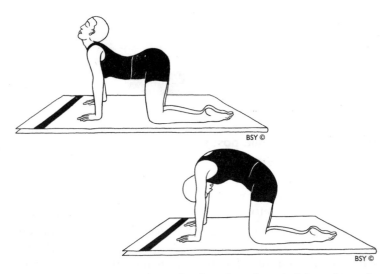

Exhale while lowering the head and stretching the spine upward.

At the end of exhalation, contract the abdomen and pull in the buttocks.

The head will now be between the arms, facing the thighs. Hold the breath for 3 seconds, accentuating the arch of the spine and the abdominal contraction.

This is one round.

Breathing: Perform the movement breathing as slowly as is comfortable. Aim at taking at least 5 seconds for both inhalation and exhalation.

Duration: Perform 5 to 10 full rounds for general purposes.

Awareness: Physical – on the movement of the spine from top to bottom, and on the breath synchronized with the movement.

Spiritual – on swadhisthana chakra.

Benefits: This asana improves the flexibility of the neck, shoulders and entire spine. It induces deep breathing. It gently tones the female reproductive system, giving relief from menstrual cramps and leucorrhoea.

Practice note: Do not bend the arms at the elbows. Keep the arms and thighs vertical throughout.

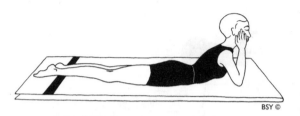

BSY ©

Makarasana (crocodile pose)

Lie flat on the stomach.

Raise the head and shoulders and rest the chin in the palms of the hands with the elbows on the floor.

Keep the elbows together for a more pronounced arch to the spine. Separate the elbows slightly to relieve excess pressure on the neck.

In makarasana the effect is felt at two points: the neck and the lower back. If the elbows are too far in front, tension will be felt in the neck; if they are drawn too close to the chest, tension will be felt more in the lower back. Adjust the position of the elbows so that these two points are equally balanced. The ideal position is when the whole spine is equally relaxed.

Relax the whole body and close the eyes.

After some time, again become aware of the body and surroundings, and gently and smoothly release the posture.

Breathing: Natural and rhythmic, or practise inhaling, moving the awareness up along the spine from the tail bone to the neck and exhaling, bringing the awareness back down from the neck to the tail bone. Feel the breath moving up and down the spine. This will quickly activate the healing energies in this area.

For lower back pain due to tension, concentrate on this area and feel it expanding and relaxing with every inhalation and exhalation.

Duration: For as long as is comfortable.

Awareness: Physical – with concentration on the lower back, and relaxing the whole body, and on the breathing process. Spiritual – on manipura chakra.

Contra-indications: Those with back conditions, such as exaggerated lumbar curve, should not practise this asana if any pain is experienced.

Benefits: This asana is very effective in lower back pain. It is practised for extended periods of time as it encourages the vertebral column to resume its normal shape and releases compression of the spinal nerves. People with lung ailments should practise this simple asana regularly with breath awareness as it allows more air to enter the lungs.

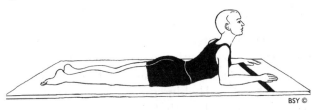

Saral Bhujangasana (easy cobra pose)

Lie flat on the stomach with the forehead resting on the floor, the legs straight, feet together, and the soles of the feet facing up.

Bend the arms and place the forearms on the floor with the palms downward on each side of the head. The fingertips point forward, but are in line with the crown of the head. The forearms and elbows are close to the body. Relax the whole body.

Raise the head, shoulders and chest by bringing the upper arms to the vertical position.

The elbows, forearms and hands will remain on the floor. Relax in the position for a comfortable length of time and then slowly lower the body.

This is one round.

Breathing: Inhale while raising the head, shoulders and chest, exhale while lowering to the floor. Breathe normally in the final position.

Duration: Hold the position for 3 to 4 minutes as a static pose or practise up to 5 rounds as a dynamic pose.

Awareness: Physical – on the sensation in the arms and shoulders, on relaxing the back, and on the breath.
Spiritual – on swadhisthana chakra.
Benefits: This asana strengthens the arms and shoulders and is especially good for stiff backs.

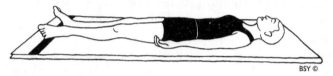

BSY ©

Shavasana (corpse pose)

Lie flat on the back with the arms about 15 cm away from the body, palms facing upward. A thin pillow or folded cloth may be placed behind the head to prevent discomfort. Let the fingers curl up slightly.

Move the feet slightly apart to a comfortable position and close the eyes.

The head and spine should be in a straight line.

Make sure the head does not fall to one side or the other.

Relax the whole body and stop all physical movement.

Become aware of the natural breath and allow it to become rhythmic and relaxed.

After some time, again become aware of the body and surroundings, and gently and smoothly release the posture.

Breathing: Natural and relaxed, or begin to count the breaths from number 27 backwards to zero. Mentally repeat, "I am breathing in 27, I am breathing out 27, I am breathing in 26, I am breathing out 26", and so on, back to zero.

If the mind wanders and the next number is forgotten, bring it back to the counting and start again at 27. If the mind can be kept on the breath for a few minutes, the body will relax.

Duration: According to time available. In general, the longer the better, although a minute or two is sufficient between asana practices.

Awareness: Physical – first on relaxing the whole body, then on the breath.

Spiritual – on ajna chakra.

Benefits: This asana relaxes the whole psycho-physiological system. It should ideally be practised before sleep; before, during and after asana practice, particularly after dynamic practices such as surya namaskara; and when the practitioner feels physically and mentally tired. It develops body awareness. When the body is completely relaxed, awareness of the mind increases, developing pratyahara.

Practice note: Do not move the body at all during the practice as even the slightest movement disturbs the practice.

A personal mantra may be repeated with every inhalation and exhalation.

For maximum benefit, this technique should be performed after a hard day's work, before evening activities, or to refresh the body and mind before sitting for meditation, or just before sleep.

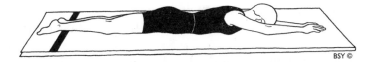

Advasana (reversed corpse pose)

Lie on the stomach.

Stretch both arms above the head with the palms facing downward. The forehead should be resting on the floor.

Relax the whole body in the same way as described for shavasana.

If there is difficulty breathing or a sense of suffocation is experienced, a pillow may be placed under the chest.

After some time, again become aware of the body and surroundings, and gently and smoothly release the posture.

Breathing: Natural and rhythmic. The number of breaths may be counted as in shavasana while gently pushing the abdomen against the floor.

Duration: For relaxation in the treatment of ailments, it should be performed for as long as is comfortable. Before or during an asana session, a few minutes is sufficient.

Awareness: Physical – on relaxing the whole body, and on the breath.

Spiritual – on ajna or manipura chakra.

Benefits: Recommended for those with slipped disc, stiff neck and stooping figure.

Practice note: Mantra may also be synchronized with the breath as in shavasana.

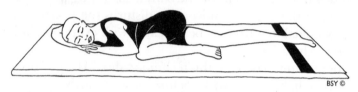

BSY ©

Matsya Kridasana (flapping fish pose)

Lie on the stomach with the fingers interlocked under the head. Bend the left leg sideways and bring the left knee close to the ribs.

The right leg should remain straight.

Swivel the arms to the left and rest the left elbow near the left knee.

Rest the right side of the head on the crook of the right arm, or a little further down the arm for more comfort.

Relax in the final pose and, after some time, change sides. This position resembles a flapping fish.

After some time, again become aware of the body and surroundings, and gently and smoothly release the posture.

Breathing: Normal and relaxed in the static pose.

Duration: Practise this asana for as long as is comfortable on both sides. It may also be used for sleeping and resting.

Awareness: Physical – on relaxing the whole body, and on the breath.

Spiritual – on manipura chakra.

Benefits: This asana stimulates digestive peristalsis. It relieves sciatic pain by relaxing the nerves in the legs. People for whom the practice of forward bending asanas is not recommended may practise matsya kridasana as a counterpose after backward bending asanas. It relaxes tension in the perineum. The bent knee and the head may be supported on a pillow for further comfort.

Sukhasana (easy pose)

Sit with the legs straight in front of the body.

Bend one leg and place the foot under the opposite thigh.

Bend the other leg and place the foot under the opposite thigh.

Place the hands on the knees in chin or jnana mudra.

Keep the head, neck and back upright and straight, but without strain. Close the eyes.

Relax the whole body. The arms should be relaxed and not held straight.

Benefits: Sukhasana is the easiest and most comfortable of the meditation postures. It can be utilized without ill effect by persons who are unable to sit in the more difficult meditation postures. It facilitates mental and physical balance without causing strain or pain.

Practice note: Sukhasana is a relaxing posture which may be used after extended periods of sitting in siddhasana or padmasana.

Although sukhasana is said to be the simplest meditation posture, it is difficult to sustain for long periods of time unless the knees are close to the ground or on the ground. Otherwise most of the body weight is supported by the buttocks and backache develops. The other meditation asanas create a larger and therefore steadier area of support.

Variation: For those who are extremely stiff, sukhasana may be performed sitting cross-legged with a belt or cloth tied around the knees and lower back.

Hold the spine upright.

85

Concentrate on the physical balance and equalizing the weight on the right and left side of the body. A light, spacey feeling may be experienced.

While maintaining the posture, place the hands on the knees in chin or jnana mudra.

Ardha Padmasana (half lotus pose)

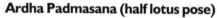

Sit with the legs straight in front of the body.

Bend one leg and place the sole of the foot on the inside of the opposite thigh.

Bend the other leg and place the foot on top of the opposite thigh.

Without straining, try to place the upper heel as near as possible to the abdomen. Adjust the position so that it is comfortable.

Place the hands on the knees in either chin or jnana mudra. Keep the back, neck and head upright and straight. Close the eyes and relax the whole body.

Contra-indications: Those who suffer from sciatica or knee problems should not perform this asana.

Benefits: The same benefits as given for padmasana but at a reduced level.

Padmasana (lotus pose)

Sit with the legs straight in front of the body.

Slowly and carefully bend one leg and place the foot on top of the opposite thigh.

The sole should face upward and the heel should be close to the pubic bone.

When this feels comfortable, bend the other leg and place the foot on top of the opposite thigh.

Both knees should, ideally, touch the ground in the final position.

The head and spine should be held upright and the shoulders relaxed.

Place the hands on the knees in chin or jnana mudra.

Relax the arms with the elbows slightly bent and check that the shoulders are not raised or hunched.

Close the eyes and relax the whole body.

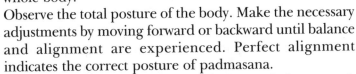

Observe the total posture of the body. Make the necessary adjustments by moving forward or backward until balance and alignment are experienced. Perfect alignment indicates the correct posture of padmasana.

Contra-indications: Those who suffer from sciatica or weak or injured knees should not perform this asana. This asana should not be attempted until flexibility of the knees has been developed through practice of the pre-meditation asanas.

Benefits: Padmasana allows the body to be held completely steady for long periods of time. It holds the trunk and head like a pillar with the legs as the firm foundation. As the body is steadied, the mind becomes calm. This steadiness and calmness is the first step towards real meditation. Padmasana directs the flow of prana from mooladhara chakra in the perineum to sahasrara chakra in the head, heightening the experience of meditation.

This posture applies pressure to the lower spine, which has a relaxing effect on the nervous system. The breath becomes slow, muscular tension is decreased and blood pressure is reduced. The normally large blood flow to the legs is redirected to the abdominal region. This activity also stimulates the digestive process.

Siddhasana (accomplished pose for men)

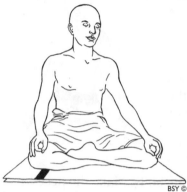

Sit with the legs straight in front of the body.

Bend the right leg and place the sole of the foot flat against the inner left thigh with the heel pressing the perineum (the area midway between the genitals and anus).

Bend the left leg. Push the toes and the outer edge of the left foot into the space between the right calf and thigh muscles. If necessary, this space may be enlarged slightly by using the hands or temporarily adjusting the position of the right leg. Place the left ankle directly over the right ankle so that the ankle bones are touching and the heels are one above the other.

Press the pubis with the left heel directly above the genitals. The genitals will therefore lie between the two heels.

If this last position is too difficult, simply place the left heel as near as possible to the pubis.

Grasp the right toes and pull them up into the space between the left calf and thigh.

Again adjust the body so that it is comfortable.

Sit on top of the right heel. This is an important aspect of siddhasana. Adjust the body until it is comfortable and the pressure of the heel is firmly applied.

The legs should now be locked, with the knees touching the ground and the left heel directly above the right heel. Make the spine erect and feel as though the body is fixed on the floor.

Place the hands on the knees in jnana, chin or chinmaya mudra.

Close the eyes and relax the whole body.

Contra-indications: Siddhasana should not be practised by people with sciatica.

Benefits: Siddhasana directs the energy from the lower psychic centres upward through the spine, stimulating the brain and calming the entire nervous system.

This posture redirects blood circulation to the lower spine and abdomen, toning the lumbar region of the spine, the pelvis and the abdominal organs, and balancing the reproductive system and the blood pressure.

Practice note: Siddhasana may be performed with either leg uppermost. Many people experience discomfort due to the pressure applied where the ankles cross each other. If necessary, place a folded cloth or piece of sponge between the legs at this point. At first the pressure at the perineum may be uncomfortable to maintain, but with practice this will be eased.

Siddha Yoni Asana (accomplished pose for women)

Sit with the legs straight in front of the body.

Bend the right leg, placing the sole of the foot flat against the inner left thigh and the heel firmly against the groin.

Adjust the body position so that there is comfortable pressure of the right heel.

Bend the left leg and wedge the left toes down into the space between the right calf and thigh.

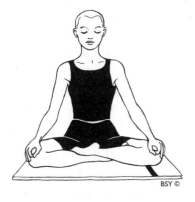

Grasp the toes of the right foot and pull them up into the space between the left calf and thigh.

The left heel is above the right heel and may exert a light pressure against the pubic bone.

Again adjust the position so that it is comfortable.

Ensure that the knees are firmly on the ground.

Make the spine fully erect and straight as though it were planted solidly in the earth.

Place the hands on the knees in chin or jnana mudra. Close the eyes and relax the whole body.

Contra-indications: As for siddhasana.

Benefits: As for siddhasana.

Swastikasana (auspicious pose)

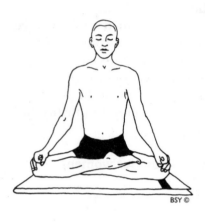

Sit with the legs straight in front of the body.

Bend the left knee and place the sole of the left foot against the inside of the right thigh so there is no contact between the heel and the perineum.

Bend the right knee and place the right foot in the space between the left thigh and calf muscle so that there is no contact between the heel and the pubis.

Grasp the toes of the left foot and pull them up into the space between the right calf and thigh.

Adjust the position so that it is comfortable. The knees should be firmly on the floor.

Straighten the spine. Place the hands on the knees in chin or jnana mudra.

Variation: Sit with the legs straight in front of the body.

Bend the left leg and place the sole against the inside of the right thigh.

Similarly, bend the right leg and place the heel of the right foot on the floor in front of the left foot with the sole resting against the left shin. The heels will now be one in front of the other.

The hands may be placed on the knees in chin or jnana mudra, or they may be placed in the lap.

Close the eyes and relax the whole body.

Contra-indications: Swastikasana should not be performed by people with sciatica.

90

Benefits: Swastikasana is a healthy position to sit in, especially for those suffering from varicose veins, tired and aching muscles or fluid retention in the legs.

Practice note: This is the easiest classical meditation asana and is a simplified version of siddhasana.

PRE-PRANAYAMA PRACTICES AND PRANAYAMA

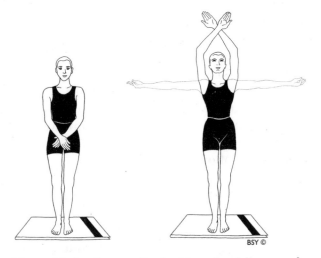

Bandha Hasta Utthanasana (locked hand raising pose)

Stand erect with the feet together and the arms by the sides. Relax the whole body and balance the body weight equally on both feet.

Cross the wrists in front of the body.

Slowly raise the arms above the head, keeping the wrists crossed, and at the same time bend the head slightly backward and look up at the hands.

Spread the arms out to the sides so that they form a straight line at shoulder level.

Hold the position, then reverse the movement, re-crossing the wrists above the head.

Lower the arms straight down so that they are once again in the starting position, and look forward.

Repeat the process 10 times.

Breathing: For beginners – inhale raising the arms, exhale while spreading them out to the sides, inhale while re-crossing the wrists above the head, and exhale while lowering the arms.

For more experienced practitioners – inhale while raising the arms and inhale more deeply while spreading them out to the sides. Exhale while re-crossing the wrists above the head and exhale more deeply while lowering the arms.

Awareness: On the stretch in the arms and shoulders, the expansion of the lungs, and on the breath synchronized with the movement.

Benefits: This asana rectifies round shoulders and removes stiffness from the shoulders and upper back. The deep, synchronized breaths improve breathing capacity. This asana also influences the heart and improves blood circulation. The whole body, especially the brain, receives an extra supply of oxygen.

Jnana Mudra (psychic gesture of knowledge)

Assume a comfortable meditation posture.

Fold the index fingers so that they touch the inside root of the thumbs. Straighten the other three fingers of each hand so that they are relaxed and slightly apart.

Place the hands on the knees with the palms facing down. Relax the hands and arms.

Chin Mudra (psychic gesture of consciousness)

Chin mudra is performed in the same way as jnana mudra, except that the palms of both hands face upwards, with the backs of the hands resting on the knees.

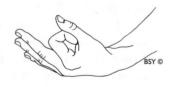

Relax the hands and arms.

Sequence: One of these two mudras should be adopted whenever practising meditation, unless otherwise specified.

Benefits: Jnana mudra and chin mudra are simple but important psycho-neural finger locks which make meditation asanas more powerful.

Practice note: The effect of chin and jnana mudras is very subtle and it requires great sensitivity on the part of the practitioner to perceive the change in consciousness established. With practice, however, the mind becomes conditioned to the mudra and when it is adopted, the signal to enter a meditative state is transmitted.

Hridaya Mudra (heart gesture)

Sit in any comfortable meditation asana with the head and spine straight.
Place the tips of the index fingers at the root of the thumbs, as in chin and jnana mudras, and join the tips of the middle and ring fingers to the tips of the thumbs. The little finger remains straight.
Place the hands on the knees with the palms facing upward.
Close the eyes and relax the whole body, keeping it motionless.

Duration: This practice may be performed for up to 30 minutes.

Awareness: Physical – on the breath in the chest area.
Spiritual – on anahata chakra.

Benefits: This mudra diverts the flow of prana from the hands to the heart area, improving the vitality of the heart. The middle and ring fingers relate directly to nadis connected with the heart, while the thumb closes the pranic circuit and acts as an energizer, diverting the flow of prana from the hands to these nadis. Hridaya mudra is therefore beneficial for the heart. It is very simple and may be used safely and easily, even in acute situations. The heart is the centre of emotion. Hridaya mudra helps to release pent-up emotion and unburden the heart. It may be practised during emotional conflict and crisis.

Natural breathing

This is a simple technique which introduces practitioners to their own respiratory system and breathing patterns. It is very relaxing and may be practised at any time. Awareness of the breathing process itself is sufficient to slow down the respiratory rate and establish a more relaxed rhythm.

Technique

Sit in a comfortable meditation posture or lie in shavasana and relax the whole body.

Observe the natural and spontaneous breathing process.

Develop total awareness of the rhythmic flow of the breath.

Feel the breath flowing in and out of the nose.

Do not control the breath in any way.

Notice that the breath is cool as it enters the nostrils and warm as it flows out.

Observe this with the attitude of a detached witness.

Feel the breath flowing in and out at the back of the mouth above the throat.

Bring the awareness down to the region of throat and feel the breath flowing in the throat.

Bring the awareness down to the region of the chest and feel the breath flowing in the trachea and bronchial tubes.

Next, feel the breath flowing in the lungs.

Be aware of the lungs expanding and relaxing.

Shift the attention to the ribcage and observe the expansion and relaxation of this area.

Bring the awareness down to the abdomen. Feel the abdomen move upward on inhalation and downward on exhalation.

Finally, become aware of the whole breathing process from the nostrils to the abdomen and continue observing it for some time.

Bring the awareness back to observing the physical body as one unit and open the eyes.

Abdominal (or diaphragmatic) breathing

Abdominal or diaphragmatic breathing is practised by enhancing the action of the diaphragm and minimizing the action of the ribcage. The diaphragm is a domed sheet of muscle that separates the lungs from the abdominal cavity and, when functioning correctly, promotes the most efficient type of breathing. It is the effect of the diaphragm rather than the diaphragm itself that is experienced as the stomach rises and falls, but sensitivity will come with practice. During inhalation the diaphragm moves downward, pushing the abdominal contents downward and outward. During exhalation the diaphragm moves upward and the abdominal contents move inward.

Movement of the diaphragm signifies that the lower lobes of the lungs are being utilized. The proper use of the diaphragm causes equal expansion of the alveoli, improves lymphatic drainage from basal parts of the lungs, massages the liver, stomach, intestines and other organs that lie immediately beneath it, exerts a positive effect on the cardiac functions and coronary supply, and improves oxygenation of the blood and circulation.

Abdominal breathing is the most natural and efficient way to breathe. However, due to tension, poor posture, restrictive clothing and lack of training, it is often forgotten. Once this technique again becomes a part of daily life and correct breathing is restored, there will be a great improvement in the state of physical and mental wellbeing.

Technique

Place the right hand on the abdomen just above the navel and the left hand over the centre of the chest.

Observe the spontaneous breath without controlling it in any way. Let it be absolutely natural.

Let the abdomen relax. Do not try to force the movement in any way.

Do not expand the chest or move the shoulders.

Feel the abdomen expanding and contracting.

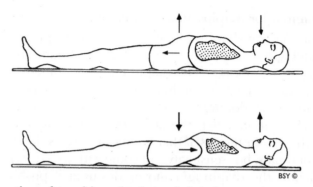

Continue breathing slowly and deeply.

Inhale while expanding the abdomen as much as is comfortable, without expanding the ribcage.

At the end of the inhalation, the diaphragm will be compressing the abdomen and the navel will be at its highest point.

On exhalation, the diaphragm moves upward and the abdomen moves downward.

At the end of the exhalation, the abdomen will be contracted and the navel compressed towards the spine.

The right hand will move up with inhalation and down with exhalation. The left hand remains almost still.

Continue for a few minutes.

Relax any effort and once again watch the spontaneous breathing pattern.

Bring the awareness back to observing the physical body as a whole. Be aware of the surroundings and gently open the eyes.

For cancer patients: This is the correct method of breathing all the time for everyone, but it is especially recommended in cancer of the upper abdominal organs (liver, gall bladder, stomach and pancreas etc.), any cancer with fluid collection in the abdomen and any cancer with secondaries in the liver.

Thoracic breathing

Thoracic breathing utilizes the middle lobes of the lungs by expanding and contracting the ribcage. It expends more energy than abdominal breathing for the same quantity of air exchange. It is often associated with physical exercise and exertion, as well as stress and tension; when combined with abdominal breathing, it helps the body to obtain more oxygen. However, the tendency in many people is to continue this type of breathing instead of abdominal breathing long after the stressful situation has passed, creating bad breathing habits and continued tension.

Technique

Sit in a meditation posture or lie in shavasana and relax the whole body.

Maintain unbroken awareness of the natural breath for some time, concentrating on the sides of the chest.

Discontinue any further use of the diaphragm and begin to inhale by slowly expanding the ribcage.

Feel the movement of the individual ribs outward and upward, and be aware of this expansion drawing air into the lungs.

Expand the chest as much as possible.

Exhale by relaxing the chest muscles. Feel the ribcage contracting and forcing the air out of the lungs.

Breathe slowly and deeply through the chest with total awareness. Do not use the diaphragm.

Continue thoracic breathing for a few minutes, pausing slightly after each inhalation and exhalation.

Relax any effort and once again watch the spontaneous breathing pattern.

Bring the awareness back to observing the physical body as a whole. Be aware of the surroundings and gently open the eyes.

Yogic breathing

Yogic breathing combines the previous two techniques. It is used to maximize inhalation and exhalation. Its purpose is to gain control of the breath, correct poor breathing habits and increase oxygen intake.

It may be practised at any time and is especially useful in situations of high stress or anger for calming the nerves. However, while its inclusion in a daily yoga program will correct and deepen natural breathing patterns, yogic breathing itself should not be performed continually.

Technique

Sit in a meditation posture or lie in shavasana and relax the whole body.

Inhale slowly and deeply, allowing the abdomen to expand fully.

Try to breathe so slowly that little or no sound of the breath can be heard.

Feel the air reaching into the bottom of the lungs.

At the end of abdominal expansion, start to expand the chest outward and upward allowing the ribs to expand fully.

Feel the air filling the whole of the lungs.

This completes one inhalation.

The whole process should be one continuous movement. There should be no jerks or unnecessary strain. The breathing should be like the swell of the sea.

Now start to exhale.

First, relax and allow the chest to contract downward and then inward.

Next, allow the diaphragm to push upward and toward the chest.

Without straining, try to empty the lungs as much as possible by drawing or pulling the abdominal wall as near as possible to the spine.

The entire movement should be harmonious and flowing.

Hold the breath for a few seconds at the end of exhalation.

This completes one round of yogic breathing.

At first perform 5 to 10 rounds and slowly increase to 10 minutes daily.

Relax any effort and once again watch the spontaneous breathing pattern.

Bring the awareness back to observing the physical body as a whole. Be aware of the surroundings and gently open the eyes.

Nadi Shodhana Pranayama (psychic network purification)
Hand position: Nasagra Mudra (nosetip position)

Hold the fingers of the right hand in front of the face.

Rest the index and middle fingers gently on the eyebrow centre. Both fingers should be relaxed.

The thumb is above the right nostril and the ring finger above the left. These two digits control the flow of breath in the nostrils by alternately pressing on one nostril, blocking the flow of breath, and then the other.

The little finger is comfortably folded.

When practising for long periods, the elbow may be supported in the palm of the left hand, although care is needed to prevent chest restriction.

Technique I: Preparatory practice

Stage I: Sit in any comfortable meditation posture, preferably siddha/siddha yoni asana or padmasana.

Keep the head and spine upright.

Relax the whole body and close the eyes.

Practise yogic breathing for some time.

Adopt nasagra mudra with the right hand and place the left hand on the knee in chin or jnana mudra.

Close the right nostril with the thumb.

Inhale and exhale through the left nostril 5 times.

The rate of inhalation/exhalation should be normal.

Be aware of each breath.

After completing 5 breaths, release the pressure of the thumb on the right nostril and press the left nostril with the ring finger, blocking the flow of air.

Inhale and exhale through the right nostril 5 times, keeping the respiration rate normal.

Lower the hand and breathe 5 times through both nostrils together.

This is one round.

Practise 5 rounds or for 3 to 5 minutes, making sure that there is no sound as the air passes through the nostrils.

Practise until this stage is mastered before commencing the next stage.

Stage 2: Begin to control the duration of each breath.

Count the length of the inhalation and exhalation through the left, right and both nostrils. Breathe deeply without strain.

While inhaling, count mentally, "1, Om; 2, Om; 3, Om", until the inhalation ends comfortably.

While exhaling, simultaneously count, "1, Om; 2, Om; 3, Om". Inhalation and exhalation should be equal.

Practise 5 rounds or for 3 to 5 minutes, making sure that there is no sound as the air passes through the nostrils.

Extension: Notice that the length of the breath will spontaneously increase after some days of practice.

When the count reaches 10 without any strain, go on to technique 2.

Contra-indications: Nadi shodhana is not to be practised while suffering from colds, flu or fever.

Benefits: Technique 1 increases awareness of and sensitivity to the breath in the nostrils. Minor blockages are removed and the flow of breath in both nostrils becomes more balanced. Breathing through the left nostril tends to activate the right brain hemisphere; breathing through the right nostril activates the left hemisphere. The long, slow, balanced breathing of stage 2 has profound effects, calming and balancing the energies.

Practice note: Both nostrils must be clear and flowing freely. Mucous blockages may be removed through the practice of neti. If the flow of breath in the nostrils is unequal, it may be balanced by practising padadhirasana as a breath balancing technique (Refer to *Asana Pranayama Mudra Bandha,* a Yoga Publications Trust publication.)

Beginners should be familiar with abdominal and yogic breathing before taking up nadi shodhana pranayama.

Technique 2: Alternate nostril breathing

In this technique the basic pattern of alternate nostril breathing is established.

Stage 1: Begin with equal inhalation and exhalation, using the ratio 1:1.

Close the right nostril with the thumb and inhale through the left nostril.

At the same time count mentally, "1, Om; 2, Om; 3, Om", until the inhalation ends comfortably. This is the basic count.

Breathe deeply without strain.

Close the left nostril with the ring finger and release the pressure of the thumb on the right nostril. While exhaling through the right nostril, simultaneously count, "1, Om; 2, Om; 3, Om". The time for inhalation and exhalation should be equal.

Next, inhale through the right nostril, keeping the same count in the same manner.

At the end of inhalation, close the right nostril and open the left nostril. Exhale through the left nostril, counting as before.

This is one round.

Practise 5 to 10 rounds.

Extension: After one week, if there is no difficulty, increase the length of inhalation/exhalation by one count.

Continue to increase the count in this way until the count of 10:10 is reached.

Do not force the breath in any way. Be careful not to speed up the counting during exhalation to compensate for shortage of breath. Reduce the count at the slightest sign of discomfort.

Stage 2: After perfecting the above 1:1 ratio, it may be changed to 1:2.

Initially halve the length of the inhalation. Inhale for a count of 5 and exhale for a count of 10.

Repeat on the other side.

This is one round.

Practise 5 to10 rounds.

Extension: During the ensuing months of practice, continue extending the breath by adding one count to the inhalation and two to the exhalation, up to the count of 10:20.

When this technique can be performed with complete ease, move on to technique 3.

Contra-indications: Stage 2 of technique 2 begins the process of introversion, which is not recommended for a depressed or withdrawn person. The extension of stage 2, involving longer counts, is not recommended for people with heart problems.

Benefits: Technique 2 gives more pronounced balancing of the breath and the brain hemispheres. It has calming effects and relieves anxiety, improves concentration and stimulates ajna chakra.

The ratio 1:1 in stage 1 establishes a calming rhythm for the brain and heart, assisting people with cardiovascular and nervous disorders specifically, and stress-related conditions generally.

As the count is extended, the breath slows down. The respiration becomes more efficient because the air flow is smoother and less turbulent. This ratio helps people with respiratory problems.

The ratio 1:2 in stage 2 gives profound relaxation. The heartbeat and pulse rate slow, and blood pressure reduces. The extension of count should be built up slowly.

Ujjayi Pranayama (the psychic breath)

Sit in any comfortable meditation asana.

Close the eyes and relax the whole body.

Take the awareness to the breath in the nostrils and allow the breathing to become calm and rhythmic.

After some time, transfer the awareness to the throat.

Feel or imagine that the breath is being drawn in and out through the throat and not through the nostrils, as if it is taking place through a small hole in the throat.

As the breathing becomes slower and deeper, gently contract the glottis so that a soft snoring sound, like the breathing of a sleeping baby, is produced in the throat. If practised correctly, there will be a spontaneous contraction of the abdomen, without any effort being made.

Both inhalation and exhalation should be long, deep and controlled.

Practise yogic breathing while concentrating on the sound produced by the breath in the throat.

The sound of the breath should be audible to the practitioner alone.

Extension: When this breathing has been mastered, fold the tongue back into khechari mudra (see below).

If the tongue becomes tired, release it, while continuing the ujjayi breathing. When the tongue is rested, again fold it back.

Duration: Begin with 10 breaths and slowly increase to 5 minutes for general benefits.

As an adjunct to meditation or mantra repetition, practise for 10 to 20 minutes.

Contra-indications: People who are too introverted by nature should not perform this practice.

Benefits: Ujjayi is classified as a tranquillizing pranayama and it also has a gentle heating effect on the body. This practice soothes the nervous system and calms the mind. It has a profoundly relaxing effect at the psychic level. It helps to relieve insomnia and may be practised in shavasana just before sleep. It slows down the heart rate and is useful for people suffering from high blood pressure. It is very useful for those with a weak heart or breathing difficulty as it improves oxygenation of the blood and reduces the work load on the heart.

For cancer patients: People with cancer of the throat area (larynx, pharynx, tonsils, soft palate, base of the tongue etc.) may find it too difficult to practise ujjayi pranayama with or without khechari mudra as the breathing passage of the area may already be partially blocked due to cancer, or the muscles may be weak.

Ujjayi is especially recommended in lung cancer, cancer of the throat area (larynx, pharynx, tonsils, soft palate, base of the tongue etc.) when possible, any cancer with secondaries in the lungs, any cancer with water logging of the lungs and any cancer with fluid in the pleural cavity. Ujjayi breathing in the frontal psychic passage is useful in breast cancer. Ujjayi breathing in the spinal psychic passage is useful in any cancer with secondaries in the vertebral column.

Practice note: Ujjayi may be performed in any position, standing, sitting or lying. Those suffering from slipped disc or vertebral spondylitis may practise ujjayi in vajrasana or makarasana with the awareness moving up and down the spinal column with inhalation and exhalation.

Relax the face as much as possible. Do not contract the throat too strongly. The contraction should be slight and applied continuously throughout the practice.

Khechari Mudra (tongue lock)

Sit in any comfortable meditation pose, preferably padmasana or siddha/siddha yoni asana, with the head and spine straight and the hands in chin or jnana mudra. Relax the whole body and close the eyes.

Fold the tongue upward and backward, so that the lower surface lies in contact with the upper palate.

Stretch the tip of the tongue backward as far as is comfortable.

104

Do not strain.

Perform ujjayi pranayama.

Breathe slowly and deeply.

Hold the tongue lock for as long as possible without straining.

At first there may be some discomfort and ujjayi pranayama may irritate the throat, but with practice it will become more comfortable.

When the tongue becomes tired, release and relax it, then repeat the practice.

Duration: Practise for 5 to 10 minutes. Khechari mudra may also be performed with other yoga practices.

Awareness: Physical – on the stretch of the tongue and the light pressure against the upper palate.

Spiritual – at vishuddhi chakra.

Precaution: Discontinue this mudra if a bitter secretion is tasted. Such a secretion is a sign of toxins in the system.

Contra-indications: Tongue ulcers and other common mouth ailments will temporarily preclude performance of this practice.

Benefits: This practice reduces the sensations of hunger and thirst, and induces a state of inner calm and stillness. It preserves the vitality of the body and is especially beneficial for inner healing.

For cancer patients: Khechari mudra is contra-indicated in cancer of the tongue, soft palate and tonsils. It may be difficult in any cancer of the oral cavity in general. It is not to be practised when strong medications (chemotherapy, hormones, strong antibiotics etc.) are circulating in the body or their effects are still being experienced.

A basic yoga nidra practice may be given to a beginner by an experienced yoga teacher. Include stages 1, 3, 4, 6, 7 and 8. At appropriate time stage 2 may be introduced.

Alternately, use audio recordings available from Yoga Publications Trust.

Connecting to the self

Please start the practice with the first four stages of yoga nidra: preparation and relaxation, resolve, rotation of consciousness on body parts and breathing. Omit stage 5 (feelings and sensations) and continue with stages 6, 7 and 8 (visualization, resolve, ending the practice).

Stage 6: Visualization
1. Inner space

Ocean: Think of an ocean . . . think of a dark blue ocean and become aware of the waves. *(pause)* That ocean lies within the inner space, the chidakasha, and the rolling waves represent sleep . . . the manifesting unconscious state of your mind. *(pause)* Become aware of sleep and try to visualize this state of unconsciousness within you, like waves on an ocean. *(pause)* Above is a beautiful blue sky and below is the vast ocean with infinite waves . . . the manifesting process of unconsciousness. *(long pause)*

Well: Imagine a well, imagine a well and that you are looking into it. The well is dark and deep . . . a cylindrical tunnel into the depths of the earth. *(pause)* There is a bucket on a chain; you lower it into the well . . . and it moves into abysmal darkness . . . you can feel it on the chain, in the depths . . . but you cannot see it. *(pause)* Now pull the bucket up, up out of the darkness and into the light . . . let's lower the bucket again, but this time if you wish, you can get into the bucket, and I will lower you down and pull you up again, perfectly safely. *(pause)* Now the bucket is winding down, you are descending slowly through the light and moving into darkness . . . unknown, all-pervading darkness. *(pause)* Complete darkness and emptiness all around . . . so dark you cannot see yourself, but you can know and feel that you are. *(pause)* You descend a little further, with complete awareness that you are. *(pause)* Now I am winding you up, up through the darkness . . . and into the dim light; from the dim light into daylight and out of the well. *(pause)*

Spontaneous thought: Now ask yourself: 'What am I thinking?' . . . do not 'think' but become aware of the spontaneous thought process . . . become a witness, do not suppress any thought. *(pause)* Try to witness your thoughts and ask yourself again and again: 'What am I thinking?' *(pause)* At the same time, maintain total awareness of any thought that is passing through the visible frame of your consciousness. *(long pause)*

2. **Movement in time**: Now you are going to travel into your past, in the same way you have travelled from the past to the present . . . retracing the steps of your memory and consciousness backwards from this time. The past is part of time and time is part of your mind. Normally you walk forward in time . . . this time try and walk backwards. By remembering your past you are going into the deeper recesses of your consciousness. *(pause)*

Try to remember what happened from the present time to the time you got up this morning . . . you have to go back in time as if you were watching a film running in reverse, or if not a film, a series of slides. *(pause)* Remember back to the start of the yoga nidra, then recall what you were doing in the half hour before that. *(pause)* Remember the important objects and feelings in that time, and then keep on proceeding in half hour or one hour stages, to when you woke up. *(long pause)* Stage by stage, with full awareness, visualize and recall what you were doing, thinking and feeling. *(pause)* When you have finished, bring your mind directly back to the present. *(long pause)*

3. **Rapid image**: Bring your awareness to the present and make sure you are not sleeping, no sleeping please. I am going to name a few objects and you should try to visualize them on the levels of feeling, awareness, emotion and imagination as best you can. *(pause)* You should move as fast as I go, jumping your mind from image to image; do not waste your time concentrating on any one image, but keep moving.

Shivalingam . . . standing Christ . . . flickering candle . . . weeping willow tree . . . tall palm tree . . . car moving on a road . . . dead body burning over a fire . . . coloured clouds gathering . . . yellow clouds . . . blue clouds . . . starlit night . . . full moon . . . dog standing . . . cat reposing . . . elephant moving . . . horse racing . . . rising sun . . . setting sun . . . ocean with waves . . . shivalingam . . . standing Christ . . . a big pond with clear water . . . blue lotus . . . white lotus . . . pink lotus . . . golden spider web . . . sandy bank of a wide river . . . boat sailing on the water . . . see the ripples . . . dead body burning on a fire . . . human skeletons . . . yourself lying down without clothes . . . completely naked . . . golden cord extending from your navel into the sky . . . cross over a church . . . within the church a priest praying . . . worshipper kneeling . . . chimney smoke rising from an old house . . . a cold winter . . . a fire burning in the house . . . dawn of the day . . . temple bell ringing . . . a monk with shaven head . . . a yogi sitting in deep meditation . . . Buddha in repose . . . Christ showing compassion. *(pause)*

Resolve: Resolve, resolve, resolve . . . now you should remember your resolve and repeat it three times. *(pause)* With maximum feeling and awareness, three times. *(pause)*

Finish: Now relax all efforts and bring your attention to the natural breath, the natural breath flowing in and out of the nostrils. *(long pause)* Maintain your awareness of the breath and at the same time develop your awareness of physical relaxation. *(pause)* Awareness of relaxation . . . and awareness of your physical existence; become aware of the physical existence of your body. *(long pause)* Develop awareness of your body and visualize your body lying on the floor. *(pause)* Take your mind out and visualize the surrounding room, let your mind become completely external . . . do not open your eyes. *(pause)* You are practising yoga nidra, become aware of this fact. *(pause)* Lie quietly until your attention is completely externalized. Start moving, moving your body and stretching yourself . . . please take your time, there is no hurry. *(pause)* When you are sure that you are wide awake, sit up slowly and open your eyes. The practice of yoga nidra is now complete.

Hari Om Tat Sat

Alternative visualizations

Any one of the following visualization sequences can be substituted for the visualizations from 'Rapid Images' and completed with 'Resolve' and 'Finish' as above.

1. ***Eyebrow centre/Om***: Concentrate on the eyebrow centre. *(pause)* With the breath, see the expansion and contraction of *Om*, in a circle. *(pause)* In the eyebrow centre with the rhythm of the breath, expansion and contraction of *Om* in a circle. *(long pause)*

2. ***Golden egg***: Become aware of yourself. Find out by asking yourself: 'Am I aware of myself? Am I asleep or awake?' See your whole body from top to toe, as clearly as I see it . . . try to see your body by being outside it. Ask yourself: 'Am I this body, the body that is eventually going to die?' *(pause)* Now look to your senses, the five senses by which you know this world. Ask yourself: 'Am I these senses, the senses that die with the body?' *(pause)*
Now, try to become aware of yourself, look at the mind, the mind by which you understand yourself and the world. Ask yourself: 'Am I the mind, the mind that also dies?' *(pause)* Become aware of yourself, look at yourself and become aware of your aura . . . become aware of this. Ask

yourself: 'Am I this aura, whose existence is tied to the body?' *(pause)* Look further . . . become aware of the prana in your body. Ask yourself: 'Am I this prana?' *(pause)* Again look within and become aware of the existence of your consciousness, by which you know that you are practising yoga nidra. Ask yourself: 'Am I this consciousness? Does this consciousness still survive after the death of the body?' *(pause)*

Look within, and become aware of a golden egg in the centre of your brain . . . a golden egg, very small, very small, that is the seat of your highest consciousness. *(pause)* A golden egg, very small, that is the seat of supreme consciousness within you, at your centre . . . try to identify with it. *(long pause)* Try to see yourself as the golden egg . . . and say to yourself: 'Beyond the mind, body, senses, the karma, the nature, and everything that is physical, mental, psychic, unconscious, I am in the form of this golden egg.' *(long pause)* Say to your mind: 'I am that.' *(long pause)*

3. **Inner love visualization**: Relax your body and become aware of your heart, right in the middle of your chest. Make sure your mouth remains closed and imagine that you are breathing in and out through your heart. You should breathe deeply and be completely aware of each incoming and outgoing breath.

Imagine the air you are breathing is a golden colour . . . like mist . . . and you are taking this golden mist into your body through the heart and spreading it about inside.

Fill your body with this golden mist. Feel that every time you breathe in you are cleaning out your whole body with this mist and it is giving you many good qualities. It gives you all forms of goodness, love, honesty, cooperation, understanding, peace and happiness. As you breathe out, all the things you don't want or don't like about yourself pass out from your body: unhappiness, disobedience, anger, meanness, cruelty, dislikes . . . all these things are carried away by the golden mist. Become aware of your heartbeat. Listen to the steady sound of your heart. Imagine that in your heart the golden mist has formed into a very small golden egg. The golden egg breaks open and there in your heart, sitting on a beautiful flower, is a tiny little being, the size of your thumb. This little being is surrounded by a cloud of bright light. It is sitting very still and silently and looking at you and sending you love and happiness. Let yourself be filled by its love.

This beautiful little being is sending you so much love, and the more it gives, the brighter its light becomes. It is giving you so much love that you cannot keep it all in, you must send it out to all other people. Think of your parents and your brothers and sisters and send this love out to them. Think of all the sick, unhappy and lonely people in the world and send them this love. Think of all the people you do not like, send out the love to them. Remember your friends and send them this love. The more love you send out the more the little being in your heart fills you with love. Now become aware of the room in which you are sitting. Fill this room with the love that is within you.

PRATYAHARA AND DHARANA PRACTICES

Kaya Sthairyam

This practice is preliminary to any pratyahara or dharana (meditation) practice. The Sanskrit word *kaya* means body and *sthairyam* means steadiness or lack of movement. A steady, comfortable, motionless body induces the mind to become still and quiet. It prepares the mind to introvert, to start looking in.

Stage 1: Preparation

Sit in a comfortable meditation posture, preferably siddha/ siddha yoni asana or padmasana. Adjust your position so that you do not have to move any part of the body during the practice. Make sure the spine is erect. Head, neck and shoulders should be slightly back. Place your hands on

111

the knees in chin or jnana mudra. Close your eyes. Become aware of slow, deep breathing and count five breaths mentally.

Stage 2: Body posture

Switch your awareness to the body. Concentrate on your meditation posture. Feel your spine rising straight up from the floor, supporting the head. Be aware of the synchronized and balanced position of the arms and legs. Maintain total awareness of the body.

Stage 3: Visualization of body

Visualize your body externally as if you were seeing it in a full length mirror. See your body in the meditation posture from the front, from the back, from the right side, from the left side, from the top. See your body from all sides at one time.

Stage 4: Immobility of the body

Make a resolve that, "I will not move my body throughout the whole practice. My body will not move or shake. I will remain steady and motionless like a statue." Even if you feel an impulse to move a finger or toe, to adjust your clothing, or to scratch, try to overcome this urge. When you feel the urge to move you must say to yourself "No, I will not move any part of my body until the end of the practice."

Stage 5: Steadiness and stillness

Be aware of your physical body, of your meditation posture and of nothing else. There should be total uninterrupted awareness of the whole body. The body is perfectly steady and motionless. Develop the feeling of steadiness. Be aware of your body and steadiness. Be aware of your body and stillness. Your body is absolutely steady and still. Be aware of steadiness. Be aware of your physical body. There is no movement, no discomfort, only steadiness and stillness.

Now either proceed to the pratyahara or dharana practice of your choice or end the practice by going to the next stage.

Stage 6: Ending the practice

Get ready to end the practice. Gradually become aware of the physical body, of the meditation posture. Feel the weight of the body against the floor. Be aware of the hands resting on the knees. Be aware of the whole physical body. Be aware of the breathing. Watch the breath as it flows in and out. Take a deep breath in and chant *Om* three times.

Hari Om Tat Sat

Dharana Darshan, published by Yoga Publications Trust, is recommended for further reading.

Antar Mouna

Antar mouna can be practised in any meditation posture like padmasana, siddhasana, vajrasana or sukhasana, or, if these are not possible, in shavasana, lying down, or while seated and relaxed in a comfortable chair.

Antar mouna, particularly the earlier stages, can be practised anywhere at any time. It can even be used to calm the mind in the most unpleasant surroundings and in the midst of intense noise. If you want to include antar mouna in your daily sadhana program, the best time to practise is either late at night just before sleep, or early in the morning. At these times there will be the least noise and fewer disturbances. Try to practise for a fixed period each day for as long as you have time to spare.

Contra-indications: People with depression or other mental problems, or an inability to control the thought process consciously, should not practise antar mouna. It should also not be practised when the mind is in a pessimistic mood.

Technique
Stage I: Awareness of sense perceptions

Close your eyes and become aware of the whole body. Without moving, experience the sensation of touch. Be aware of the parts of the body that are in contact with the

113

floor, the contact points of your clothing and skin. Fix your whole attention on the sense of touch until you lose interest in it.

Then become aware of the outside environment. Be aware of all the external sounds; listen carefully with detached awareness. Do not judge, analyze or think about the sounds . . . only listen to the sounds. Focus your attention on the most prominent sound for a few minutes, then dismiss it and find another.

Now become aware of your breath. Fix your whole attention on the flow of the breath; cut off the perception of external sounds. Continue breath awareness for a few minutes. Then again direct your attention to the outside world and each and every sound. Be alert, don't introvert and become lost in thoughts.

After some minutes, again become aware of the breathing process. Forget the outer sounds; only perceive the flow of the breath.

Continue in this manner, externalizing and internalizing your awareness; sense (sound) awareness, breath awareness. Continue for as long as you have time available.

Practice note: Stage 1 of antar mouna should be practised regularly until you have developed the ability to detach yourself completely from outside activities, particularly sounds. It is possible to become so introverted that even if a telephone rings, you will not have any reaction to it. When you reach this stage, you will be ready to proceed to stage 2. This will probably take at least one month of daily practice.

Stage 2: Awareness of the spontaneous thought process

Practise antar mouna stage 1 (awareness of external sounds) for a few minutes and then proceed to stage 2.

Forget the outer world and focus your full attention on the thought processes.

Be aware of every thought. The past, figures and faces of your friends, people whom you love and hate, let them come. But remember, you don't belong to them, nor they

114

to you. You are the witness and they are passing objects.
If someone you love suddenly comes before your mind
and you go on developing the fantasy, this means that you
are attached to that thought. Attachment to a thought
produces more thoughts and creates further impressions
which your consciousness records within. Without interfer-
ing, allow your mind to think anything it wishes. Only be a
witness; try to be a detached, uninfluenced observer of all
your thoughts.

Allow all the emotions such as hatred, anger, fear, guilt,
etc. to arise and be released, but remain a witness, a seer,
separate from the emotions and thoughts.

Open the door to your conscious mind. Look inside and
remove all the useless mental debris that is accumulated there.
Then after 5 minutes or so become aware of chidakasha,
the dark space in front of the closed eyes. This is the
screen of your mind on which it is possible to see
subconscious visions. If visions arise, merely observe them
as a witness. If no visions come, continue to watch for a
few minutes, then return your awareness to the thought
process. If you experience momentary absent-mindedness,
imagine that you are looking down a long road. The road
is clear, no one is in sight. (The road is your conscious
mind.) Then someone appears on the road, you see
shadows moving. They are the shadows of your thoughts.
Continue to alternate between watching your thought
processes and the dark screen of chidakasha. Practise for
as long as you have time available.

Now get ready to end the practice. Withdraw your
awareness from the thought process. Become aware of
your physical body which is sitting in the meditation
posture. Feel your physical body from head to toe. Be
aware of the weight of the body against the floor. Feel the
hands resting on the knees. Become aware of the external
sounds. Slowly move your fingers and toes. Breathe in
deeply and chant *Om* three times.

Hari Om Tat Sat

Practice note: Stage 2 should be practised daily until you have developed the ability to remain detached and uninvolved in your thoughts.

You should proceed to stage 3 if you start having psychic visions. If you don't experience visions, you may commence the next stage when you have spent at least one month practising stage 2.

Please refer to *Sure Ways to Self Realization*, a Yoga Publications Trust publication, for more details. Audio recordings are also available for the practice of antar mouna from Yoga Publications Trust.

Ajapa Dharana One: Frontal Passage Rotation

In the practices of ajapa dharana, various psychic passages have been utilized in order to channel the awareness, the breath and the mantra. The first one, which is given here, is the frontal psychic passage which extends from the navel to the throat.

This practice comprises several stages which develop the awareness of the psychic passage. First the breath is moved up and down in a straight line from the navel to the throat and from the throat to the navel. Then the frontal psychic passage is visualized as a luminous, transparent tube. Afterwards the breath is rotated inside the psychic passage. When this has been mastered, the rotation of prana is then visualized inside the frontal passage. This is followed by rotation of the *Soham* mantra. With each stage an increasing build-up of energy inside the frontal passage is experienced and concentration becomes deeper and more one-pointed. This practice follows the principle that an awakening of energy brings about an awakening of consciousness, which makes it easier to concentrate and focus the mind on one point.

Technique
Stage 1: Preparation

Sit in a comfortable meditation asana. Ensure that the spine is straight. The head, neck and shoulders should be slightly back. Place the hands on the knees in chin or jnana mudra. Become aware of your body and meditation posture. Feel the position of the body from the top of the head to the toes. Feel the body posture becoming steady and still. Continue with total awareness of the body and of stillness.

Stage 2: Breath awareness

Switch your awareness from the body to the breath. Practise slow, deep breathing. As you breathe in, count to five. As you breathe out, count to five. Concentrate on the breathing in the throat. As you breathe in and out, feel the breath moving through the throat. As you concentrate on the rhythmic breathing in the throat, you will gradually feel the steadiness of the mind and body as a whole.

Now become aware of the breath moving from the navel to the throat. Bring your awareness to the navel. Inhale slowly in a straight line from the navel up to the throat. Then exhale slowly in a straight line from the throat down to the navel. Count to five each time you breathe in and out. Go on breathing up and down from navel to throat, throat to navel, until the breath moves along this fixed pathway easily without conscious effort. Watch the movement carefully without missing a single breath.

Stage 3: Frontal passage visualization

Leave awareness of the breath for a few moments and visualize the psychic passage between the navel and the throat, at the front of the body. See the psychic passage as a long, thin, transparent tube, connecting the navel with the throat. This tube is hollow and open at both ends, like a flute. You can blow through it from the top or the bottom. Visualize this luminous, transparent tube and move your awareness up and down along the outside surface. Try to see the entire length of the tube very

117

clearly. Take your awareness inside the tube, and move it up and down the centre, visualizing the tube from within.

Stage 4: Breath rotation inside the psychic passage

Resume your awareness of slow, deep breathing. Feel the breath moving inside the frontal passage between the navel and the throat. While inhaling, the breath ascends from the navel to the throat. While exhaling, the breath descends from the throat to the navel. Try to visualize clearly the inside of the psychic passage with the ascent and descent of each breath. Feel as if the awareness is moving together with the breath up and down the centre of the psychic passage. As the breath moves through the passage, the awareness also moves. Develop the feeling of two distinct forces, the breath and the consciousness, moving together inside the psychic pathway.

Stage 5: Rotation of prana

Intensify awareness of the breath and the consciousness moving together inside the psychic passage. Feel the flow of breath and consciousness, ascending and descending together through the psychic passage. Gradually become aware of a third force, the pranic force, which is moving together with the breath and the consciousness. It requires a subtle awareness to perceive the flow of prana moving with the breath. The breath moves in the form of wind or air, while prana moves in the form of energy. Become aware of the energy, the prana, moving with the breath. It is actually this flow of prana or energy between the navel and the throat which creates the psychic passage, in the same way that flowing water creates a stream.

Be aware of the prana moving with the breath inside the psychic passage. Visualize the thin, sparkling stream of energy, of prana, which flows upward from the navel to the throat as you breathe in and downward from the throat to the navel as you breathe out. Watch carefully and try to experience the movement of prana inside the psychic passage. At first you may need to use your imagination, but with practice you will spontaneously feel

118

a powerful current of energy flowing up and down the psychic passage. Be aware of the movement of prana with each breath.

Stage 6: Rotation of Soham

Now leave awareness of the prana and intensify awareness of the breath. Listen carefully to the subtle sound of each breath as it moves up and down the frontal passage. The inherent sound of the breath is the mantra *Soham*. As you breathe in, hear the mantra *So* and as you breathe out, hear the mantra *Ham*. This *Soham* mantra is not separate from the breath. You are not repeating it verbally. It is already going on within the breath each time you breathe. You must become aware of it, that is all.

Listen carefully while inhaling and try to hear the sound *So-o-o-o*. While exhaling hear the sound *Ham-m-m-m*. Concentrate totally on the process of breathing together with the mantra of the breath, which is *Soham*. As the breath moves, the sound moves with it.

Be aware of the movement of the breath and the vibration of the *Soham* mantra inside the frontal passage. Concentrate your entire awareness inside the psychic passage. There should be no other thought, vision or experience. Try to feel that the entire breathing process is taking place inside the psychic passage only. As the breath becomes more and more subtle, the vibration of the mantra also becomes more subtle. Gradually you will begin to perceive this process as a psychic movement within the frontal passage. The dimension of your consciousness will change as the mind becomes totally absorbed in the psychic movement of the breath and the mantra. Nothing else exists outside of the psychic passage, the breath and the mantra.

Stage 7: Ending the practice

Now get ready to end the practice. Withdraw your awareness from the frontal passage and the mantra. Change over to normal breathing. Again become aware of your physical body which is sitting in the meditation posture. Feel your physical body from head to toe. Be aware of the weight of the body against the floor. Feel the hands resting on the knees. Slowly move your fingers and toes. Breathe in deeply and chant *Om* three times.

Hari Om Tat Sat

Dharana Darshan, published by Yoga Publications Trust, is recommended for further reading. Audio recordings are also available for this practice from Yoga Publications Trust.

Trataka

The word *trataka* means steady gazing. The practice of trataka involves gazing at a point or object without winking or blinking the eyes. It is a method of focusing the eyes, and in turn the mind, on one point to the exclusion of all others. When the object is external, the practice is called *bahya drishti trataka* and when internal, *antar drishti trataka.*

When the same object is continuously seen, the brain becomes habituated and soon stops registering that object. This is true for any other sensory stimulus, sound, touch, taste, etc. and the mind tends to turn off and falls asleep. The key point, however, is to stay alert and aware. When the mind is isolated from all the sense organs and associated mental processes such as thoughts, memories, emotions etc. and still kept alert, then spiritual consciousness emerges. The practice of trataka is used in one form or another in all religions as a means of spiritual upliftment.

The object of trataka can be almost anything that attracts your attention and holds it. You must decide what is most suitable for you. The following are some commonly used objects: candle flame, the symbol of Om, a cross, the moon, water, a black dot, one's *ishta deva* (chosen deity), a *yantra* (specific geometrical symbol).

Benefits: Trataka relieves eye strain, insomnia, stress and anxiety. It improves concentration and memory.

Precaution: Trataka must be practised on a still object. Avoid a flickering flame or moving water. Trataka on a flame or any other very bright object should not be continued for more than two months at a stretch. Take a break of a few days and then resume again. Trataka on the sun can be harmful to the eyes.

People with myopia (short-sightedness) severe enough to warrant glasses should retain their glasses while practising trataka on a flame.

Contra-indications: In major eye problems such as retinal detachment, macular dysfunction, advanced diabetic or hypertensive retinopathy, advanced cataract, etc. trataka should not be practised regularly. People suffering from glaucoma or epilepsy should not practise trataka.

Trataka stage 1: Bahya Drishti (external gazing)
Technique 1: Trataka on a candle flame

Place the candle in the correct position (at eye level and an arm's length away) in front of you and light it. The room should be dark and without any direct strong breeze. Sit in a comfortable meditation posture. Close your eyes. Concentrate on steadiness of the body. Feel your entire body becoming steady and motionless like a statue. Be aware of absolute steadiness and stillness. Make a resolve not to move your body during the practice. If you move even slightly, your concentration will be broken.

Open your eyes and gaze at the candle flame. Focus your gaze at the tip of the wick, without straining. Your eyes should be completely relaxed. If you try too hard to focus on the flame, there will be more tension and movement of the eyes. Consciously relax the eye muscles. Try not to blink or move the eyes in any way. Keep your focus steady as you gaze at the wick of the candle flame.

Let your whole awareness be on the candle flame and wick. If thoughts come, let them. Be aware of them and then gently bring your whole awareness back to the candle flame. See the candle flame clearly. Though your vision is focused on one point you can see the whole candle. Be aware of the shape and colours of the candle flame. Allow your attention to be completely absorbed in the flame. There is only the flame.

If you need to close your eyes, then do so and rest them for a few moments. During this practice tears should not fall, so close your eyes before you feel this will happen. When they are rested, then again open them and focus at the tip of the wick. Continue with the practice in this way.

Technique 2: Trataka with breath awareness

While gazing at the candle flame become aware of your breath. Begin to practise ujjayi pranayama. Let the tongue slip back into khechari mudra. Now imagine that you are drawing your breath from the candle flame to the eyebrow centre and back to ajna chakra at the centre of the head. When you exhale, imagine that the breath flows from ajna chakra, pierces the eyebrow centre and returns to the candle flame. You must split your awareness so that you are simultaneously aware of the candle flame and the movement of the breath. The eyes should remain steady and relaxed throughout.

Continue in this way, breathing in and out while you feel or imagine the breath moving backwards and forwards from the candle flame through the eyebrow centre to ajna chakra and back again to the flame. Be aware of the candle flame, the breath and the subtle sound of the ujjayi breath. Intensify your awareness of this pathway between the candle flame and ajna chakra. Feel you are connecting these points, the flame, *bhrumadhya* (eyebrow centre) and ajna chakra. Be aware of every breath. Continue in this way for some time.

Trataka stage 2: Bahya-Antar Drishti (outer-inner gazing)
Technique: Trataka on a candle flame

Sit in any comfortable meditation posture. Place the hands on the knees and close the eyes. Move your awareness through the body and relax the body completely. Feel the whole body becoming steady and still.

Now become aware of the position of the legs. Feel that the legs are comfortable and the hands are relaxed. Become aware of the hands and arms. Feel that the arms are relaxed and still. Become aware of the whole back. The back is straight but without tension. Bring your awareness to the front of the body. Check that there is no tension in the abdomen or chest. Become aware of the head. There should be no tension between the eyebrows or around the jaw.

Next become aware of the whole body together. Be aware of every part of the body. Feel the stillness of the body. There is no movement in any part of the body. The whole body is comfortable and still. Intensify this awareness of stillness throughout the whole body. Experience stillness and quietness.

Now open the eyes and gaze intently at the candle flame. Try not to wink or blink. Continue gazing steadily for three minutes. Then close your eyes and try to visualize the after-image of the candle flame at the eyebrow centre. Gaze at the inner image in the same way that you gazed at the external candle flame. This is a combination of trataka on the external object and the internal after-image.

See somewhere in chidakasha a tiny, luminous, coloured dot. Gaze steadily at the dot. It is similar to a small grain of wheat, rice or barley in shape, but the colour changes from moment to moment. The colour depends on how long you have been gazing at the candle flame. After one minute the colour will be black, white or dull brown. After about five minutes, the colour of the dot will be bright red.

If the image is not clear at first, just be aware of whatever you can see. Keep the eye muscles relaxed throughout the practice; this helps you to get a clear inner image. If the image is moving, follow it and gently bring it back to the eyebrow centre. Take a few moments to steady the image. If the image fades or disappears, do not worry; just try to recreate it again. The image will become clear and vivid as the eyes become relaxed and steady.

From moment to moment the dot becomes dimmer and suddenly disappears. All this happens within a few seconds, but you should be careful not to open the eyes. Even if the psychic point disappears, keep your eyes closed. Again try to assemble the psychic awareness and recollect the psychic point. In a few seconds the internal object will reappear and when it reappears, it will have a different colour altogether. Continue gazing at the internal point with the help of your inner perception, your inner vision, your inner eye. It will grow fainter and fainter and still fainter, and then it will disappear. Do not open your eyes. Assemble your awareness again. Recollect the internal point and see it come once more before your vision.

Thus this psychic point appears, disappears, reappears, disappears, again reappears, becomes dim, disappears, reappears, again grows dimmer and dimmer. Ultimately it becomes absolutely black and merges with the psychic background.

This is one round. Practise one to three rounds.

Trataka stage 3: Antar Drishti (inner gazing)
Technique: Antar trataka on a candle flame

Sit in a comfortable, steady position. Close your eyes and keep them closed for the duration of the practice. Practise kaya sthairyam. Be aware of the steadiness of the whole body. Feel that the body is immovable. It is fixed to the floor, in fact, it is part of the floor. Continue to practise kaya sthairyam for a few minutes until you feel the body becoming stiff and rigid like a statue.

Now bring your awareness to bhrumadhya, at the eyebrow centre. Without creating any strain focus your total attention on the sensation between the eyebrows. Try to think of nothing else apart from the eyebrow centre. Continue in this manner until you can feel a definite sensation at this point.

Now visualize the flame of a candle at the eyebrow centre. Try to hold the image steadily. If you cannot see it, then

124

imagine it. If the image fades or disappears, you must recreate it. Maintain the inner vision of the candle flame. Go on watching it. It may vanish and reappear. Continue to recreate the image at the eyebrow centre. With practice the image should be as clear and vivid as if you were looking at it with open eyes. Hold the image of the candle flame steadily at bhrumadhya. Do not let it waver.

There should be continuous, unbroken awareness of the candle flame. Gradually let everything dissolve and just be aware of the candle flame. Try to identify, to merge your mind totally with the image. Continue in this way for as long as possible.

Then slowly let go of the image. Bring the awareness to the natural, spontaneous breath. Be aware of the slow, steady flow of the breath. Become aware of the body and your meditation posture. Listen to any sounds inside and outside the room. Breathe in deeply and chant *Om* three times. Then slowly move the body and open the eyes.

Hari Om Tat Sat

Refer to *Dharana Darshan*, published by Yoga Publications Trust, for more detail.

Mantra meditation

Om meditation

Practise kaya sthairyam. *Pause.* Become aware of your normal breath. *Pause.* Allow it to become slower and deeper. *Pause.* With the in-going breath take your awareness within the chest. Find the innermost point in your chest cavity. It is the point that your breath is touching as you breathe in. In order to identify it, allow the consciousness to flow in with the inhalation as far as the breath goes and then stay at that point. *Pause.* Once you identify that point, keep you awareness steady there and let go of breath awareness. *Pause.* Visualize a bright non-flickering jyoti or candle flame at this point. *Pause.* Now start chanting the mantra *Om* mentally, maintaining awareness of the jyoti. With every exhalation chant *Om* once. Let the *O* be long and towards the end of the exhalation complete it with *m*. Breathe in and while exhaling say *O o o o o m m*. Breathe in again and while exhaling say *O o o o o m m*. Continue at your own pace. *Pause.* Feel the vibration of the sound. *Pause.* The centre of the sound waves is at the jyoti. The ripples are travelling outward, filling up your whole body and the surroundings. *Pause.* Awareness is simultaneously on the jyoti, on the mantra *Om* and on the ripples. *Pause.* Now stop chanting the mantra. Remain aware of the jyoti and the ripples. Gradually the ripples fade away. Only the jyoti remains. Feel immense peace, harmony and joy within. *Pause.* Chant the Shanti mantras with feeling and conviction. *Pause.* Allow the image of the jyoti to dissolve. Become aware of your breath. *Pause.* Become aware of your body sitting on the ground. *Pause.* Feel the weight of the body against the floor. Be aware of one part of the body touching the other. The hands are touching the knees, the feet are touching each other or the thighs, the lips are touching each other and so on. *Pause.* Extend the awareness outside the body into your surroundings. Become aware of various sensations arising from the atmosphere around you; various sounds, fragrance, touch and perception of light or darkness. *Pause.* When your mind is fully externalized, then gradually start moving your body, rub your palms, cover the closed eyes with the warm palms for a short time and then open your eyes.

Hari Om Tat Sat

Mantra japa

The word *japa* means 'to rotate', and the practice of japa yoga involves continuous rotation of a mala, a string of 108 beads, in synchronization with a mantra. *Japa yoga* means 'union with the highest existence through rotation of consciousness'.

Of all the systems of meditation, japa is the most popular. It is a part of most religions and cultures and is applicable to everyone. It is the easiest form of meditation for those who do not have the guidance of a guru.

The technique of japa yoga is primarily meant for the awakening of psychic awareness in the average individual as well as for the spiritual aspirant. It is particularly suitable for those who have a restless, unstable mind and for all who are tamasic or rajasic by nature.

During japa one has to chant a mantra and rotate the beads of the mala. These act as a point of reference for the awareness. After a short time a rhythm is established; the movement of the mala becomes synchronized with the chanting. If one tends to fall asleep or become too involved in thoughts, the mantra repetition and movement of the mala will become uncoordinated or stop altogether. This will gently remind the practitioner to return to the practice.

While practising japa, thoughts will arise and these must be witnessed and not suppressed. Most thoughts that arise during meditation are very superficial and they must be cleared away to allow the deeper tensions of the mind to manifest. After steady, regular practice of japa, the mind will be overwhelmed by the mantra and less interested in the monotonous patterns of thought. Mental turmoil will subside and a balanced, harmonious mind will result.

When the mind has become still and you have become deeply absorbed in your mantra, a vision or unexpected thought may suddenly manifest. This represents a deeper problem which you must witness without any involvement. If you can do this, it may be all that is needed to remove it. If you have this experience, understand that you are cleansing the mind and are now beginning to penetrate its deeper layers. Let your thoughts flow and let the japa process continue simultaneously. Sometimes awareness of thinking will become keen and at other times awareness of the mantra will predominate. There is an alternate awareness of wavering and concentration, fluctuation and unification; this must happen.

One should never wish to be completely free of thoughts in meditation. It is impossible to be totally aware of only the japa or the mantra. Along with the mantra and the actual

127

practice of japa, thoughts will come; fluctuations must take place, memories must return. This is natural, and if it does not happen, you can be sure that you have a mental block somewhere and you must get rid of it. So, along with the mantra you can practise antar mouna, the art of witnessing the thought process.

Japa techniques

There are many different techniques of japa or mantra repetition, but they all fall into one of the following categories.

Baikhari japa is audible japa. The mantra can be chanted as loudly as you wish. This is the most suitable form of japa for beginners and people with disturbed minds. When one feels depressed, tense, angry or unhappy, this is one of the most effective methods of making the mind peaceful and harmonized. It is the practice for those who are dull, of wavering tendencies or of a restless nature. It is a very powerful practice, particularly when a large group of people chant together. The whole atmosphere is charged with positive vibrations. Audible japa should be practised for a few months by all beginners, and those who practise more advanced techniques will benefit by doing a little baikhari before their other japa. Baikhari japa can be practised with the eyes open.

Upanshu japa is whispering japa. In this form the lips are moved, but they create no loud or external sound. Only the practitioner can hear the mantra. This stage leads from simple baikhari japa to the more subtle manasik japa, and it is also useful in situations where environmental factors prevent one from practising baikhari. Whispering japa is the best form for those who want to practise hours of japa at a time. The practice of upanshu japa can be done with the eyes half closed.

Manasik is mental japa. No sound is uttered and the lips do not move. This is the most subtle form of japa and is the practice for those with a steady mind which is reasonably free of thoughts. If you do manasik japa with a disturbed mind, you will most likely fall asleep or become lost in the thought processes. If practised in a calm state of mind, manasik is the best form of japa to delve deeper into the mind. It is said by the sages and scriptures that steady and devoted practice of manasik japa is enough to lead one to enlightenment. It should always be practised with the eyes closed.

Likhit japa involves writing the mantra on paper hundreds of times in red, blue or green ink. The letters should be as small as possible and written with the utmost care, concentration and sense of beauty and proportion. The smaller the letters the greater is the concentration. Likhit japa is always combined with manasik japa. Each time the mantra is written it should be simultaneously repeated silently.

Combining the techniques

It is best to commence japa practice with baikhari, whether the mind is calm or tense. If the mind is tense, loud japa will pacify and relax the mind. If you are calm, you can quickly transfer to upanshu or manasik japa.

If you are doing manasik japa and the mind is wandering too much or becoming drowsy, you should immediately transfer to baikhari. When you have established control over the mind, you can return to manasik japa.

Which mantra and how to use it

The best mantra to use for japa is a personal mantra which has been given by a guru. If you do not have such a mantra, it is perfectly safe to use the universal mantra *Om*. Once you have begun to use a mantra, do not change it unless you have been practising with *Om* or *Soham* and a guru gives you a personal mantra.

Japa is best practiced in a steady meditation asana such as padmasana or siddhasana/siddha yoni asana. If possible, the aspirant should face north or east while practising. Use a rudraksha or tulsi mala of 108 beads with a sumeru for your guru mantra. Let the mala rest on the ring finger of your right hand. Use only the middle finger and thumb of the right hand for rolling the beads; the index and little fingers should not touch the beads. The right hand with the mala can either rest on the right knee or be held in front of the centre of the chest. The mantra should be chanted rhythmically and with clear pronunciation and intensity of feeling. The mantra must be synchronized with the movement of the mala. Each time you repeat the mantra move one bead of the mala. Do not cross the sumeru, the terminal bead, while rolling the beads. Turn the mala around when you come to the sumeru. Pronounce each letter of the mantra correctly and distinctly. Do not repeat it too fast or too slowly. Chant quickly if the mind is disturbed and slowly if the mind is more relaxed. Do not wish for any worldly objects while doing japa. Feel that your heart is being purified and the mind is becoming steady by the power of the mantra. Carry on the current of japa mentally all the time, whatever work you may be engaged in.

Japa can be practised at any time in any place, although it is best to practise at a regular time every day, either early in the morning or before sleeping at night. The mala should not be visible to others. Keep it in a cloth or silk bag when it is not in use. A japa mala should not be worn. If you want to practise while travelling to and from work, or in a place where there are other people, do not use your mala. Never practise for show; your spiritual practices should not be revealed to anyone or they will lose their power. Keep your guru mantra a secret; never disclose it to anyone.

A brief set of instructions for a more advanced variation of japa is given below.

Om chanting

Sit in a comfortable meditative posture. Relax the body and close your eyes.

Start to chant *Om* aloud. With every utterance of *Om* move one bead of your mala. *Om* chanting and rotation of the mala must be synchronized.

Try to be completely aware of the *Om* chanting and feel the vibrations of the mantra resonating through your whole being. At the same time do not forget to rotate your mala.

Continue in this manner for as long as possible (at least 10 minutes).

Then stop chanting aloud, continue to rotate the mala and take your awareness to the pulse at the eyebrow centre. When you can distinctly feel this pulse, synchronize it with mental (manasik) repetition of the mantra and rotation of the mala.

Be aware of the internal sound of *Om* at the eyebrow centre, vibrating in harmony with the pulse.

Continue in this manner for about 10 minutes, ending the practice as you complete the round of mala rotation.

Sit quietly for some moments with the awareness at either the eyebrow centre or at the heart centre. Observe what you are experiencing at that moment; the sensations, thoughts, emotions, feelings, memory, visions, or whatever. Finish by chanting *Om* aloud 3 times.

Hari Om Tat Sat

Practice note: For this practice you can choose any pulse centre for concentration, but the eyebrow centre is particularly recommended. Other useful places for pulse concentration are the heart, the throat and the navel.

Sure Ways to Self-realization and *Meditation from the Tantras*, published by Yoga Publications Trust, are recommended for further reading.

3: Learning to Cope

6

Medical Treatment

Once cancer is detected, its *grade* and *stage* can be determined. Grade means the extent of the abnormality of the cancerous cell (for example, if the cancerous cells are completely unlike their original form and are arranged in a very disorganized pattern, then the cancer is a higher grade, whereas if the cells differ only slightly from the normal original cell and are relatively neatly arranged, then the cancer is lower grade). Stage is a term that describes how far the cancer has progressed. It takes into account how big the primary tumour is, whether it has spread to lymph nodes, and whether it has metastasized (spread to distant parts of the body). For example, a small tumour with no lymph node involvement or metastasis would be considered at an earlier stage than a large tumour involving lymph nodes and other organs.

Some (but not all) cancers start off as subtle cellular changes that are described as *carcinoma in situ*. Carcinoma in situ is more easily treatable.

Early detection of cancer

The earlier the cancer is detected, the better the chance of cure.

Carcinoma of the breast can sometimes be detected by conducting a self-examination of the breasts. It is recommended that all women check their breasts every month just after the menstrual period. Put the hand flat on the breast and examine it systematically. Feel for a lump or a portion of firm-to-hard tissue. Repeat the procedure on the other side. Women with a family or personal history of breast cancer should discuss detection with their doctor. In some countries, regular clinical examination by a doctor is recommended. Mammogram (a special form of x-ray) is the best way of detecting breast cancer. In many countries women over the age of 50 are advised to have a mammogram every two years.

Cancer of the cervix is one cancer which is relatively easy to prevent, as very early pre-cancerous cellular changes can usually be detected. These changes are curable and are detected by a simple clinical procedure called a Papanicolaou (Pap) smear test. While recommendations vary between countries, in general all women should have a test at least every two years from around the age of first sexual intercourse until old age. Unfortunately there are no screening tests that are considered reliable for the early detection of ovarian cancer – it often remains difficult to detect until it is considerably advanced. (Pelvic examination by a doctor is sometimes performed, but is insensitive in detecting the early changes of ovarian cancer.)

Any non-healing ulcer or other doubtful lesion in the mouth must be medically attended to for early detection of oral cavity cancers.

For the early detection of bowel cancer, recommendations vary between countries. However, regular check-ups by a doctor that may include abdominal and digital rectal examination can sometimes be of assistance. Another screening test often offered to middle-aged or elderly people is regular (e.g. yearly) examination of the faeces for blood. In people at high risk (such as those who have a family history of bowel cancer) regular colonoscopy is often recommended. In this procedure a camera is introduced via the anus into the bowel. A biopsy can be performed on any visible abnormal lesions.

Prostate specific antigen (PSA) and digital rectal examination are often advised at regular intervals for all men above 50 years of age for the detection of prostate cancer.

Recommendations vary between countries and depend on the individual's circumstances.

All the above recommendations apply to people without any symptoms. Anyone who develops symptoms (such as a lump in the breast, odd vaginal discharge or abnormal vaginal bleeding, rectal bleeding or change in bowel or bladder habit) should see a doctor to have their specific symptoms investigated thoroughly.

Any such symptoms of unwellness should be attended to rather than ignored.

Conventional treatment of cancer

Oncology, the science that deals with cancer, treats cancer in three ways: surgery, chemotherapy and radiotherapy, and in addition hormone therapy. The site, type and stage of the cancer decide the plan of treatment.

Surgery: The first line of treatment is often surgical removal of the cancerous mass along with a small margin of normal tissue to ensure that no visible remnant of cancer is left behind in the body. (The removed portion is examined in a laboratory to ensure that, if possible, the surgical margins are clear of even microscopic portions of the cancer.) When indicated, the neighbouring (regional) lymph nodes are also removed. Sometimes, however, surgery is not possible or practical. The cancer may not be accessible to surgery, it may be too widely disseminated at the time of diagnosis, or the person may not be fit to undergo surgery. In some such cases surgery may be either preceded or replaced by either chemotherapy or radiotherapy or both.

Advocates of surgical treatment believe that surgery takes care of the major part of the enemy and that any part still remaining in the body can then be dealt with by other means. By removal of the tumour, the body's resources are also spared from constant depletion by the tumour.

Though surrounded by controversy, by and large, surgery is an accepted form of treatment for many cancers, particularly when the cancer has not yet metastasized. Surgery is sometimes also used palliatively – this means that surgery does not help cure the cancer, but it helps relieve symptoms such as excruciating pain. Surgery is often followed by chemotherapy or radiotherapy or both – again this depends upon the cancer and the individual's general health, circumstances and personal choice.

Chemotherapy: In chemotherapy, drugs that kill cells are administered. The rapidly dividing cancer cells are particularly sensitive to the effects of chemotherapeutic drugs. Their effects are extremely strong, affecting the whole body. As well as cancer cells, some types of normal cells are destroyed. Depending on the type of chemotherapy, these can particularly include the inner lining of the digestive tract, blood-forming cells in the bone marrow, hair follicles and sex glands (ovary/testis). The person receiving chemotherapy is likely to experience loss of appetite, nausea, vomiting, reduced blood cell formation leading to anaemia and impaired immune function, loss of hair, and fatigue, to name just some of the side effects. Fortunately, most of these side effects are temporary. The cells of the ovaries and testes, however, can undergo permanent damage in a person who has received chemotherapy. Therefore, an expert must be consulted both before undertaking chemotherapy and, for those who have chemotherapy before their child bearing years, before planning to have a child.

Radiotherapy: In radiotherapy ionizing radiation is directed at *the affected area* from an external source (a machine outside the body) or from an internal source (in which radioactive material is placed inside the body near the cancer cells, for example inside the vagina.) Radiotherapy affects all the cells with which it comes into contact, but cancer cells are more sensitive to its effects. Although the side effects of radiotherapy are generally much less severe than those of chemotherapy, they still occur. For many people the side effects are mild, but they can be more severe sometimes. They may include tiredness, loss of appetite or a burn on the affected area similar to a bad sunburn. Hair loss of the

138

treated area, and damage to the bone marrow, causing reduced immune function, can also occur.

Both chemotherapy and radiotherapy are administered with the aim of killing as many cancer cells as possible. Like surgery, they may be intended to be either curative or palliative. Chemotherapy and/or radiotherapy may be used in conjunction with surgery, or as the sole line/s of therapy.

The growth of certain types of cancers is affected by hormones: for example, *some* breast cancers are dependent on oestrogen, and prostate cancer on testosterone. In such cases blocking the action of the hormone with medication can be a part of the treatment A similar effect may be achieved by surgical removal of the gonad, but this is now uncommon in the developed world.

Conventional Treatment of Cancer

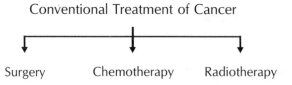

Surgery   Chemotherapy   Radiotherapy

Side effects of conventional treatments

The modern medical approach to cancer treatment is highly offensive and ruthless on the enemy, the cancerous cells. This takes its toll on the normal cells of the body. Along with the cancerous cells the normal cells also undergo the destructive actions of the various conventional treatments. With the advancement of technology these treatments are becoming more selective to cancer cells and better able to spare the normal cells. Nonetheless, conventional cancer treatment is not easy to endure. Yet, regardless of the strong side effects, complications and high expense, these treatments yield the best results. All other therapies basically work alongside, assisting rather than replacing, these conventional treatments. Each person must weigh the pros and cons before deciding whether to accept or refrain from these treatments. A lot depends upon the stage of the disease, overall physical health, personal choice and, in some cases, social as well as financial status. If the decision is taken in favour of all or some aspects of conventional treatment, then the passage can be made as smooth as possible by using yoga and other complementary systems. If the decision is made against conventional treatments, then yoga can complement alternative treatment methods.

USING YOGA TO PREPARE FOR AND COPE WITH CONVENTIONAL CANCER TREATMENTS

Surgery

Preparation for surgery: Keep the mind relaxed and focused on what needs to be done. Have a firm belief that the chosen treatment is the most beneficial for you. Find a surgeon in whom you can wholeheartedly place your trust. Practise a few simple asanas, pranayamas such as nadi shodhana or bhramari (refer to the practice sections), yoga nidra and a pratyahara or dharana practice of your choice regularly to establish and maintain the body and mind in overall good health. This improves the chances of successful outcome of the surgery.

On the day of surgery: Mantra japa, yoga nidra or breath awareness should be practised continuously for as long as possible. Mantras create a protective and healing atmosphere. Have no fear. Visualize the mantras creating a protective shield around you (refer to the practice section at the end of this chapter). Yoga nidra and breath awareness keep the mind relaxed and focused. Yoga nidra with healing visualizations is particularly recommended. Let your thoughts stay focused on the idea 'I am in the best hands and I will be cured'. A relaxed, focused and trusting mind allows the secretion of helpful chemicals that complement the healing process. If your family or friends chant prayers and healing mantras for you, so much the better.

Side effects of surgical treatment: The most common side effects are pain, fatigue and debility after surgery. Other difficulties can be nausea, vomiting, restricted movement,

140

and scarring. All but the last one are generally transient, and will pass away.

For the management of these symptoms, refer to chapter 8.

Chemotherapy and radiotherapy

Getting ready for chemotherapy or radiotherapy: Prepare the body for the treatment. Because it may not be possible to eat and drink well during the treatment, it is important to prepare the body by having a highly nutritious diet. The diet should be rich in protein, calories, vitamins and minerals. Eat nutritious, easily digestible food particularly a day or two prior to the treatment to minimize gas, constipation or diarrhoea. Each person should follow the diet that is suited to their natural constitution. Ensure good hydration. Aim to have the skin and hair in optimum condition. Attend fully to any potential focus of infection in the body (such as a cut or scratch). The treatment can temporarily depress the immune system, and any infection pre-existing in the body could flare up in the post-treatment period. Adequate rest is vital as this improves the body's coping capacity. Practise light asanas to strengthen the body. Practise pranayama regularly to improve the energy.

Prepare the mind for the treatment by helping it to relax. Yoga nidra is the most important practice to meet this need. It produces profound relaxation at the physical level, the conscious and subconscious mental levels and the emotional level. When the mind is totally relaxed, then the gates to the subconscious and unconscious mind open, releasing many suppressed past impressions. As this extra luggage is off-loaded, the relaxation deepens. The biochemistry of the body becomes conducive to repair and regeneration during states of relaxation, joy and contentment. During physical and mental relaxation the energy expenditure is curtailed. This conserved energy is then available for healing processes.

Yoga nidra is not simply a relaxation technique. Julie Friedeberger (see Appendix), a yoga practitioner who healed herself of breast cancer in 1993 and has been a yoga teacher

141

working with people with cancer since 1999, describes yoga nidra thus:

- It creates an inner environment conducive to the transformation of attitudes.
- It helps us to overcome fears, anxieties and insecurities.
- It awakens *sakshi,* the witnessing consciousness.
- It helps us develop detachment.
- It releases our samskaras.
- It teaches us to let go.

The practice section at the end of this chapter outlines yoga nidra, giving practical guidance for its use in promoting healing.

It is also important to review the decision to undergo chemotherapy or radiotherapy. Each person has the right to change that decision if they so decide. Make sure that the benefits are clearly understood and that the therapy is being accepted in spite of its limitations and hazards. Once the decision to undergo this treatment is made, believe totally that it is going to help, and wholeheartedly accept it. Practise meditation techniques such as ajapa japa or trataka regularly. This will prepare the mind to make the right decision and stick to it with certainty.

Before, during and just after chemotherapy or radio-therapy: Whilst waiting for the therapy, practise breath awareness, or mantra japa, or yoga nidra. Keep the mind focused on cheerful and optimistic thoughts. If fearful or negative thoughts arise, try to end them and substitute something positive. Practise yoga nidra during the actual administration of medication or radiation and also later while you are resting. Visualize how the treatment is fighting the cancer. Yoga nidra with healing visualizations is also very beneficial. Refer to the practice section for guidance. Alternatively, do mantra japa (repetition) continuously and feel the sound vibrations of the mantra healing your body.

The Mahamrityunjaya mantra (see the practice section for chapter 7) can be chanted by the person undergoing treatment or by family members and friends for the restoration of health. It can also be chanted throughout the period of sickness. In ashrams and centres of the Satyananda Yoga tradition around the world, this mantra is chanted on Saturday evenings for the health and wellbeing of all. Anyone can tune in by chanting the mantra 108 times wherever they are or join the group at the nearest centre.

Side effects of chemotherapy: Nausea, vomiting, loss of appetite, diarrhoea, acidity, indigestion and gas, constipation alternating with diarrhoea, fatigue and weakness, insomnia, hair loss and pigmentation of the skin are common side effects. For management of these symptoms, refer to chapter 8.

Side effects of radiotherapy: Depending on the area being treated, pain, nausea, loss of appetite, fatigue and weakness, insomnia, hair loss and pigmentation of the overlying skin are possible side effects. With newer, more precise technology in radiation oncology these side effects are minimized today.

For the management of these symptoms, refer to chapter 8.

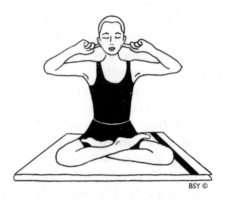

BSY ©

Bhramari Pranayama (humming bee breath)
Technique I

Sit in a comfortable meditation asana, preferably padmasana or siddha/siddha yoni asana, with the hands resting
on the knees in jnana or chin mudra.

Close the eyes and relax the whole body.

The lips should remain gently closed with the teeth slightly
separated throughout the practice. This allows the sound
vibration to be heard and felt more distinctly.

Raise the arms sideways and bend the elbows, bringing
the hands to the ears. Use the index or middle finger to
plug the ears or the flaps of the ears may be pressed
without inserting the fingers.

Bring the awareness to the centre of the head, in the
middle of the brain, and keep the body absolutely still.

Inhale through the nose.

Exhale slowly and in a controlled manner while making a
deep, steady humming sound like that of the black bee.

---

*The following practices follow on from those given in chapter 5. It is expected that
the practitioner will have some experience of the chapter 5 practices before
continuing to this stage. Only practices mentioned for the first time in chapter 6
are covered in this next section.

The humming should be smooth, even and continuous for the duration of the exhalation. The sound should be soft and mellow, making the front of the skull reverberate. At the end of exhalation, the hands can be kept steady or returned to the knees and then raised again for the next round. The inhalation and exhalation should be smooth and controlled. This is one round.

Variation: Nadanusandhana Asana (exploration of sound pose)

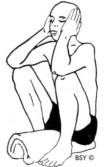

Sit on a rolled blanket with the heels drawn up to the buttocks. Place the feet flat on the floor with the knees raised and the elbows resting on the knees. Plug the ears with the thumbs, resting the other four fingers on the head. This position gives increased stability without strain when practising for long periods of time as a preparatory practice for nada yoga, which uses subtle sound vibration to attune practitioners with their true nature. In this position, continue the practice as for bhramari.

Awareness: Physical – on the humming sound within the head and on the steady, even breath.

Spiritual – on ajna chakra.

Duration: 5 to 10 rounds is sufficient in the beginning, then slowly increase to 10 to 15 minutes. In cases of extreme mental tension or anxiety, or when used to assist the healing process, practise for up to 30 minutes.

Time of practice: The best time to practise is late at night or in the early morning as there are fewer external noises to interfere with internal perception. Practising at this time awakens psychic sensitivity. However, bhramari may be practised at any time to relieve mental tension.

Contra-indications: Bhramari should not be performed while lying down. People suffering from severe ear infections should not practise this pranayama.

145

Benefits: Bhramari relieves stress and cerebral tension, and so helps in alleviating anger, anxiety and insomnia, increasing the healing capacity of the body. It strengthens and improves the voice. Bhramari induces a meditative state by harmonizing the mind and directing the awareness inward. The vibration of the humming sound creates a soothing effect on the mind and nervous system.

Yoga nidra with healing visualization

1. Healing with cosmic energy: Start the yoga nidra practice with the first four stages (preparation and relaxation, resolve, rotation of awareness on body parts, and breathing) as usual. Stage 5 (feelings and sensations) can be omitted. Then go on to stage 6 given below. Another option is to include a brief visualization just before the following stage.

Stage 6: Connecting with cosmic prana

Withdraw your mind and become aware of chidakasha, the space in front of your closed eyes. *Pause.* Imagine before you a transparent screen through which you can see infinite space, a space that extends as far as the eyes can see. *Pause.* Visualize a golden ball of light, gentle and very beautiful, in this dark vast space of chidakasha. *Pause.* Feel that as you breathe in, a ray of this golden light is lovingly touching the point between your two eyebrows, stimulating it and entering your body. As you breathe out that light spreads to all the parts of your body. As you breathe in, a ray from the golden light caresses you and enters your body through the port of the eyebrow centre. As you breathe out it spreads all through your body. With every breath your body glows more brightly. Continue with the practice. *Long pause.* This shining light in front of your closed eyes is the cosmic prana. You are connected to cosmic energy with your breath. You are breathing in nourishing, rejuvenating, healing prana and allowing it to permeate your whole being. *Long pause.* Now allow this light to flow to the weak areas of your body one by one.

Breathe in and visualize the light entering ajna chakra, the eyebrow centre. Breathe out and direct this golden light to flow towards the cancerous growth. This light is compressing, dissolving and removing the undesirable growth. It is completely restoring the health in the affected area. *Long pause.* Now start directing the light to a second area, say, where you are experiencing pain. Allow the light to remove the pain and heal the area. *Long pause.* Now move to a third area of suffering, say, digestive difficulties and direct the healing energy to the digestive system. Go on dealing with every area in the same manner. *Long pause.* Now allow the golden light to fade away gradually from your chidakasha and from within your body. *Pause.*

Repeat your resolve or sankalpa three times with full conviction. *Pause.* Become aware of your body. *Pause.* Become aware of your natural breath.

End the practice in the usual manner by gradually externalizing the awareness and moving the body (stage 8).

2. Healing with mantra energy: Start the yoga nidra practice with the first four stages (preparation and relaxation, resolve, rotation of awareness on body parts and breathing) as usual. Stage 5 (feelings and sensations) can be omitted. Then go on to the next stage given below. Another option is to introduce the mantra in stage 4 (breathing). Every act of breathing in and out is accompanied by mental mantra chanting.

Stage 6: Awakening mantra energy

Take your awareness to bhrumadhya, the centre between the two eyebrows. Let your awareness become steady, without any strain, at this point. *Pause.* While maintaining your awareness at the eyebrow centre, chant the mantra *Om* mentally, repeatedly, at your own speed and rhythm. *Long pause.* Feel the vibration at bhrumadhya. Feel the vibration of the mantra *Om* reverberating and spreading throughout your body and around you. See the vibrations

147

as a form of silvery blue ripples originating at the eyebrow centre and filling up your whole being. *Pause.* Visualize these ripples condensing at the outer periphery around your body and forming a strong shield. *Pause.* Feel that the mantra *Om* is removing everything that is harmful within and around you and is providing a protective shield for you. Under the influence of this divine power your body is healing completely and finding new vigour to fight against the disease. *Long pause.* Now cease chanting the mantra *Om*. Continue experiencing the shield, the vibrations and their effect. *Pause.*

Now let go of this experience. Repeat your resolve or sankalpa three times with full conviction. Shift your awareness from the eyebrow centre and become aware of your body. *Pause.* Become aware of your natural breath.

End the practice in the usual manner by gradually external-izing the awareness and moving the body (stage 8).

Yoga nidra during or after chemo/radiotherapy

Start the yoga nidra practice with the first four stages (preparation and relaxation, resolve, rotation of awareness on body parts and breathing) as usual. Stage 5 (feelings and sensations) can be omitted. Then go on to the next stage as given below.

Stage 6: Activating inner prana

Become aware of your whole body. Your total awareness is on your body. Visualize your body in the form of an empty shell. The body is seen as having an outer boundary of skin and nothing inside, hollow. *Pause.* Now visualize the cells of your immune system as golden luminous particles travelling all over the empty space of your body. They represent your inner strength, your prana. *Pause.* Visualize the diseased area, the cancer affected area, as black in colour. *Pause.* Visualize the medicine (or radiation) as luminous green particles entering your body and starting to move inside. Green luminous particles are the messengers of peace and healthy growth. *Pause.* Visualize the green and the golden particles travelling hand in hand towards the black area. See them converging upon and encircling this dark area. *Pause.* Visualize the golden immune cells attacking and defeating the black tumour cells with the support of the friendly green particles of chemo-medicine (or radiation). *Pause.* In this war there are casualties on both sides which are seen as red dots. Gradually the black tumour area starts shrinking in size. *Pause.* The cancerous area is being attacked and removed till the last remnant is taken care of. *Pause.* The two friends, the golden and green particles, are now rejoicing in their victory. The green particles takes leave of the golden ones and depart. The golden particles thank the green particles profusely and bid farewell to them. *Pause.* Visualize the green particles leaving and the golden immune cells happily travelling all over your body. *Long pause.*

Repeat your resolve or sankalpa three times with full conviction. Become aware of your whole body lying on the floor. Restore normal awareness of the body. *Pause.* Become aware of the natural breath.

End the practice in the usual manner by gradually externalizing the awareness and moving the body (stage 8).

Mantra Meditation
Protective shield of mantra

Practise kaya sthairyam as instructed in the practice section for chapter 5. *Pause.* Become aware of your normal breath. *Pause.* Allow it to become slower and deeper. *Pause.* Take your awareness to bhrumadhya, the centre between the two eyebrows. Let your awareness become steady, without any strain, at this point. *Pause.* While maintaining your awareness at the eyebrow centre, chant the mantra *Om* mentally, repeatedly, at your own speed and rhythm. *Long pause.* Feel the vibration at bhrumadhya. Feel the

149

vibration of the mantra *Om* reverberating and spreading throughout your body and around you. See the vibrations in the form of silvery blue ripples originating at the eyebrow centre and filling up your whole being. *Pause.* Visualize these ripples condensing at the outer periphery around your body, forming a strong shield. *Pause.* Feel that the mantra *Om* is removing everything that is harmful within and around you and is providing you with a protective shield. Under the influence of this divine power your body is healing completely and finding new vigour to fight against the evil. *Long pause.* Now stop chanting the mantra *Om*. Continue experiencing the shield, the vibrations and their effect. *Pause.*

Now let go of this experience. Repeat your resolve or sankalpa three times with full conviction. Shift your awareness from the eyebrow centre and become aware of your body. *Pause.* Become aware of your natural breath. *Pause.* Become aware of your body sitting on the floor. *Pause.* Feel the weight of the body against the floor. Be aware of one part of the body touching the other. The hands are touching the knees, the feet are touching each other or the thighs, the lips are touching each other and so on. *Pause.* Extend the awareness outside the body into your surroundings. Become aware of the various sensations arising in from the atmosphere around you: sounds, fragrances, touch and perception of light or darkness. *Pause.* When your mind is fully externalized then gradually start moving your body, rub your palms, cover the closed eyes with the warm palms together for a short time and then open your eyes.

Hari Om Tat Sat

7

The Helping Hand of Yoga

Up to this point we have tried to understand what cancer is. We have also tried to understand and develop ourselves, which is a continuous process. In this chapter we will try to learn and develop skills to cope with cancer. Medical science and alternative therapies are always available to us, but they are all only external help. Here, with the help of yoga, we will try to develop our own internal resources.

Changing the gunas

We have already discussed the concept that excessive accumulation of tamas is the cause of the origin of cancer. The only way to minimize tamas is to first bring in rajas and then subdue rajas by flooding it with sattwa. The whole process is called yoga, union with one's true self. There can be many different methods, but the end result is the same. As one travels on this path all the sufferings, including cancer, can be overcome and total healing can be attained. If persued with sincerity and faith, the end result is always very good. At the physical level, the cleansing happens in the body, in the organs, at the cellular level and even at the genetic level. On subtler planes, it happens at the pranic, mental and samskara levels.

We need to attack tamas from three different directions in order to eliminate its foothold: (i) yogic lifestyle, (ii) psychological attitudes, and (iii) yogic practices.

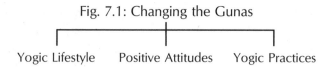

Fig. 7.1: Changing the Gunas

Yogic Lifestyle   Positive Attitudes   Yogic Practices

Yogic lifestyle: seven simple rules

The first and most basic step to reduce the strength of tamas is to make lifestyle changes. This is done by taking simple steps in daily living to ward off the effects of tamas, minimize rajas and usher in sattwa. If developed as habits when young, a yogic lifestyle can be the greatest promoter of health throughout life. Such a way of living reduces the chances of not only cancer occurring, but also other major health problems, such as obesity, diabetes, hypertension, etc. Irrespective of the stage of the disease, once lifestyle changes are made, health takes a big leap forward. There are seven simple rules for a yogic lifestyle, some of which are common rules for good health.

1. Regularity and balance
2. Moderation
3. Starting and finishing the day on a positive note
4. Living in the present moment
5. Recreation and relaxation
6. Living naturally
7. Spending time with nature.

1. Regularity and balance in daily activities is the first step in lifestyle modification. Plan a day in such a way that the normal daily activities can be maintained at their regular time. Also, while planning a day or a week, keep in mind that there needs to be a balance between physical and mental activities, work, recreation and rest, and activities for oneself and others.

After cleaning the mouth on waking in the morning, it is advisable to drink two or three glasses of plain water before doing anything else. Perform tadasana (palm tree pose), tiryaka tadasana (swaying palm tree pose) and kati chakrasana (waist rotating pose) five times each. Lukewarm water can be used, if suffering from constipation or during cold weather. One should drink at least an additional two litres of plain water during the day.

Have a regular time for waking up in the morning. Bowel movements and cleaning the body should be done at a regular fixed time daily. It is highly recommended that one rise and finish the activities necessary for cleaning the body before sunrise. Once the morning ablutions are completed, practise rejuvenating activities such as yoga, meditation, worship, taking a morning walk and sports. This is the time to be spent with and for oneself.

Breakfast, lunch, snack and dinner times should, as far as possible, be fixed. Avoid eating in between meals. Decide the menu according to the guidelines given in chapter 9 on diet. Ensure the fluid intake is adequate. Rinse the mouth properly after each meal or drink water and brush the teeth if necessary.

Minimize caffeinated beverages like tea and coffee. Completely avoid intoxicating or stimulating drinks of any kind, even if they are herbal in origin. For socializing, choose neutral herbal drinks, fresh fruit or vegetable juice, vegetable broth, lemon drinks or similar.

Prepare a work schedule and adhere to it. Develop a good work culture. Plan your work in a practical way, considering all the possibilities and obstacles. When you start implementing the plan, try to put in your best efforts, but without getting worked up about it. If you feel tension building up, immediately take a short break for two or three minutes and watch your breath or go for a stroll. If you can keep your mind off the outcome of your efforts, then tension will not build up. The trick is just to focus on how to do the job best while working and not think of the end result. Try to manage the time productively while on duty at work. Be very vigilant that time is not wasted in unproductive activities. Leave the worries of home at home. Long working hours can be broken down by short 'drink and stretch' times at regular intervals. Stretch the spine in all directions, walk, breathe in fresh air, drink a glass of water and start work again without distracting your colleagues. Include an appropriate time for socializing to link with other people. Remember to exchange a smile with your colleagues. Be sensitive to the needs of others and always be ready to offer your assistance in small ways without making people feel that they are under any obligation.

Evenings should be set aside for the family, recreation and relaxation. Do not let work or work-related thoughts occupy you at that time. Worries related to the family should be attended to at this time. It is preferable to have an early dinner. If the whole family cannot gather for dinner, then there should be a time for the family to be together at least once a day.

If you have too many things to do at work or at home, then delegate work to others, set priorities or find a solution to the situation as soon as you can. Tension builds up in proportion to the build up of pending work. Set a workable schedule and stick to it; let go of other things totally even if they seem very lucrative.

Have a regular time for going to bed. Unwind fully before retiring to bed. Analyze the day's events and your reactions to them, spending not more than fifteen minutes, meditate for a short time, usher in positive thoughts for oneself and others and fall asleep.

The schedule for holidays and weekends can include more time for recreation or socializing as the circumstances demand.

2. Moderation in every activity is the second step in lifestyle modification. Nothing should be done to extremes. Avoid too much and too little of everything, whether it is sleep, work, food, sexual activity, sensual involvement, play and entertainment or anything else. By allowing the mind to move only within a pre-selected range, we can gain control over the game of like and dislike played by the mind. We also protect ourselves from the harmful effects of over-exposure or under-exposure.

3. Starting and finishing the day on a positive note is essential to facilitate the presence of sattwa guna. Swami Niranjanananda recommends the chanting of Mahamrityunjaya mantra eleven times, Gayatri mantra eleven times and the thirty-two names of Durga three times before rising in the morning (if the body's natural calls are too urgent, then attend to them first). He says that Mahamrityunjaya mantra protects one's health at every level, Gayatri mantra opens up the intellect, and the Durga mantra removes obstacles and restores situations to a more favourable condition. These mantras can be found in the practice section after this chapter. Alternatively, one can choose any mantra, prayer, good thought or resolution to begin the day with.

At the end of the day take a quick account of the events, feelings and experiences you have had – what did you learn and was the right direction maintained? Make a brief plan for tomorrow. Erase or replace all the impressions gathered on the screen of the mind during the day by practising a short meditation. Unwind completely and allow the mind to become quiet and contented. Drift into sleep chanting a mantra of your choice, a prayer, a good thought or a resolution.

4. Live in the present moment. With each day, life begins anew. Learn from past experiences, but do not dwell on them. The past is gone, it is useless, nothing can be done about it, so let it slip away smoothly and do not hold on to it. To bring yesterday into today is to encourage tamas. So begin the day with a positive, beautiful, optimistic note. Live the day in the present moment. Be fully involved in what you are doing now. Experience the pleasant and happy moments of the present to the fullest and thank the Almighty for granting you those moments. Also experience the difficult moments of the present with full awareness. Try to find a reasonable solution and execute it to whatever extent is possible. If a satisfactory solution is not apparent, then note down the difficulty and put it aside. Allow the mind to become involved in other activities and at some later convenient time again ask the mind to search for a way out. Plan for the future constructively, but beware of slipping into unproductive day-dreaming. The only representative of eternal time that the mortal being has control over and access to is THIS MOMENT, this timeless moment.

The practice of asanas, especially when done with full awareness, pulls you right back into the present moment. It makes you intensely aware of yourself, your body with its internal organs, your mind and its thought process, and your feelings. Becoming aware of one's breathing process is another practice which serves the purpose extremely well.

5. Recreation and relaxation are often misunderstood and misused areas in life. Stretching out on a sofa, watching a film, consuming intoxicating drinks or socializing may relax the body or divert the mind from a worrying matter, but none of them can relax the mind totally. A sense of wellbeing and inner happiness is not produced by any of these activities.

Real forms of recreation are those which help us express inner thoughts and feelings directly or indirectly. It may be something physically demanding, such as sport, which can still be relaxing, as nurturing biochemicals are released in the body which produce joy, contentment and a sense of elation or euphoria. Mountaineering, gardening, sports, music, dancing, and being in natural surroundings are examples of such activities. All truly recreational activities are spontaneously relaxing.

Relaxation can also be obtained through deep sleep, meditation and yoga nidra. When the mind is totally relaxed, *samskaras*, past impressions buried in the subconscious and unconscious mind due to the constant superimposition of new ones, have a chance to surface again, thus unloading the mind. Mental relaxation then deepens. At times emotionally charged heavy impressions also become offloaded, bringing about major changes in an individual.

6. Living naturally means living in alignment and in harmony with nature. We continually receive in abundance from the natural elements, but do we give anything back? Mother Nature nurtures us all the time, so how can we nurture her? Humans are self-centred and reckless, and pay

156

little attention to the outcomes of their actions. Let us be aware of which resources we are using and the end results. We can begin with simple measures such as minimizing paper wastage, not using leather products, or synthetic non-biodegradable products, actively keeping our surroundings clean, using fuel judiciously, walking, cycling or sharing a vehicle, and avoiding preserved foods.

Another aspect of being in tune with nature is to follow its rhythm. Ayurveda describes three rhythms: *dinacharya*, the daily cycle from sunrise to sunrise, *ritucharya*, the yearly cycle of changing seasons, and *jivancharya*, the life cycle of birth, growth, stability, disease, degeneration and death. These three cycles go on and on ceaselessly. At each particular time of each cycle there are activities that are appropriate and activities to be avoided as they are unsuitable for that moment.

One should wake up one to two hours before sunrise, work and eat during the day and retire two to three hours after the sun sets, as our energy system is activated at sunrise and becomes dormant at sunset. Our hormones and digestive enzymes also wax and wane with the movement of the sun. By tuning into the sun's movements, we assist our bodily systems to function correctly and our health improves. There are appropriate activities for each time of the day. What needs to be done in the evening cannot usually be done early in the morning and so on.

Our food, clothing, temperature control in our work areas and the nature of our daily activities should change with the seasons. The best food we can eat is locally produced, seasonal and fresh. Nature always produces the food required for the season and geographical area. Similarly, our behaviour, activities and duties change with our station in life. What is appropriate for a young adult may not be desirable for a teenager or an older person.

7. Spending time with nature periodically. We are all born of Mother Nature. We derive our life energy from her and are deeply rooted in the elements of nature. It is essential to periodically spend time with her and restore our connection to her. Mountains, rivers, the ocean, gardens, meadows, lakes, trees, flowers, the breeze, sky, sun, moon and stars all arouse feelings of purity and innocence in our hearts. They represent sattwa guna. Just being in their vicinity is enough to subdue tamas. Establishing a link with them by thinking, touching, talking, nurturing and caring for them is highly beneficial.

Living in a yogic way minimizes physical, psychological and emotional stress. This helps the master controller, the neuro-endocrine axis (discussed in chapter 3) to function well, resulting in a healthy body. The immune system is assisted to work at an optimum level, minimizing the chances of illness, including cancer. Living in this way causes the least disturbance to other individuals and the environment. Exposure to various cancer risk factors is minimized, reducing the chance of genetic mutations that lead to the development of cancer occurring.

Positive psychological attitudes

Very often, the mind has a tendency towards negativity. This leads to a predominance of tamas or rajas guna. Good attitudes need to be cultivated with effort, while not so good habits and thinking patterns often come almost naturally and spontaneously. Jealousy comes spontaneously, revenge comes automatically, but compassion may need to be developed, forgiveness must be remembered again and again. Every spiritual tradition emphasizes the necessity of developing various positive psychological attitudes, which increase sattwa guna in our personality. The second step in reducing tamas and rajas gunas and increasing sattwa guna is cultivating positive attitudes.

Attitudes are responsible for our internal environment. They arise from vijnanamaya kosha, the body of wisdom. Our thoughts and behaviour are guided by our attitudes. Wrong attitudes are the source of emotional turmoil and bitter interpersonal relationships. Positive attitudes create a state of peace, harmony and balance in the mind. This, in turn, promotes healing and ushers in good health via the

158

neuro-endocrine-immune axis. Secondly, good behaviour follows good attitudes, leading to good samskaras. Good samskaras activate the maturation of the fruit of past good karmas (actions) and suppress the fructification of bad karmas. Disease is a result of bad karma. So by the law or theory of karma, good karmas and samskaras help healing in cancer.

In Patanjali's system of ashtanga yoga, purification of the mind *(chitta shuddhi)* can be attained by observing the very first two steps of raja yoga: *yama*, self-restraints or rules of conduct, and *niyama*, personal disciplines. Otherwise the mind with its impurities will not become quiet and one-pointed. There are five yamas and five niyamas. The yamas are *satya*, truth, *ahimsa*, non-violence, *asteya*, honesty or non-stealing, *brahmacharya*, establishing the mind in cosmic consciousness by restraining its associations with sense experiences, and *aparigraha*, possessing only what is really needed and letting go of what is unnecessary. The niyamas are *shaucha*, cleanliness, *santosha*, contentment, *tapas*, austerities performed to control and purify the body and mind, *swadhyaya*, observation and analysis of oneself, and *Ishwara pranidhana*, surrendering to the will of higher consciousness. Further details on the yamas and niyamas are given in the practice section at the end of this chapter.

The yamas and niyamas are the basic building blocks of every spiritual system. Most other spiritual systems recommend additional social codes of conduct and personal discipline. Only with their observation can peace, harmony and long-lasting prosperity survive. These ways of approaching life are absolutely essential for spiritual growth. When they are absent, the mindset of a human being declines into that of an animal or demon. Swami Niranjanananda recommends observing just one yama and one niyama of your choice to begin with. Choose the easiest one. Develop a clear idea of what it means to you. Observe them sincerely, honestly yet playfully. Do not allow guilt to arise when you slip. Try to sharpen the awareness gradually. Set achievable goals – go one step at a time. Review every day how are you doing in this practice. After a while observe what gives you success and what makes you slip, how to further improve your performance and how this practice has influenced your personality and life.

Initially you may find the practice challenging as it breaks many set patterns and conditionings. At the same time you will derive much satisfaction and a boost in self-esteem when you find yourself doing the right thing and not necessarily the 'in thing'. The right actions lead to a positive cycle of mental functioning – 'desire – action – experience – samskara – desire' (discussed in chapter 3). Observing the yamas and niyamas can be extended to include any quality that you want to develop.

Chapter 16 of the *Bhagavad Gita* describes the qualities of divine and demonical beings at great length. Divine, virtuous, positive qualities include: straightforwardness, giving, non-violence in thought, word and deed, truthfulness, peacefulness, compassion, modesty, forgiveness, purity, absence of hatred and absence of pride. Negative or demonical qualities limit and restrict personality development, and include: hypocrisy, anger, arrogance and self-conceit, anger and harshness, an inability to know what to do and what to refrain from and insatiable desires.

Swami Sivananda describes eighteen qualities that should be cultivated in his 'Song of eighteen ities'. The eighteen 'ities' are: serenity, regularity, absence of vanity, sincerity, simplicity, veracity, equanimity, fixity, non-irritability, adaptability, humility, tenacity, integrity, nobility, magnanimity, charity, generosity and purity.

The negative quality of finding fault with others can be added to this endless list of qualities along with the positive quality of connecting with others. Finding fault with others is actually an aspect of violence. It arises out of the basic instinct of insecurity and hence is built into our nature. In order to cover up 'something' lacking inside we look for a fault in the system outside, in a person or in the circumstance. The ego principle of our mind constantly plays this game with us. It totally clouds our intellect with wrong knowledge, leading us away from our centre and severing our connection with others. It drags us deep into the valley of tamas. This negative quality must be shunned at all costs by keeping a constant watch over ourselves – 'awareness'. As we start connecting to ourselves our concept and perception of the higher self expands. Spontaneously we start feeling a bond or oneness with others. In every act, small or big, we are thoughtful of others and the surroundings, of how our actions will affect them. *Seva*, serving others or being good to others without any selfish motive or desire for recognition helps the individual consciousness to expand and merge with cosmic consciousness.

We can gradually cultivate good qualities and get rid of the bad ones by self-observation and self-analysis. Practising the SWAN meditation is particularly helpful to bring about such changes in our personality. The habit of reviewing the day's happenings at bedtime and keeping a spiritual diary are also very helpful practices for developing or eradicating a chosen quality. Refer to the practice section at the end of this chapter for more details.

Fig. 7.2: Practices for Positive Attitudes

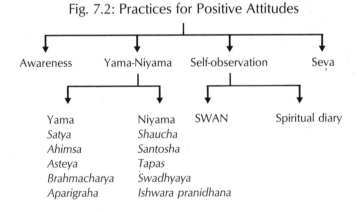

YOGA PRACTICES

The third tool in our efforts to increase sattwa guna in our personality is doing yogic practices. The word yoga means to connect with the higher self, from the Sanskrit verb *yuj*, meaning 'to unite'. *Yoga* means union of oneself with one's higher self. *Yoga vidya*, the science of yoga, deals with the process of uniting and the various means used for the purpose. The essential nature of the higher self is *sat*, eternal existence, *chit*, pure consciousness, and *ananda*, bliss. In this true nature all three gunas are in equilibrium, a state closely mimicked by sattwa predominance. The process of uniting involves minimizing tamas and rajas, thus allowing sattwa to fill up the whole being.

Depending upon the tools used, yoga is classified into many branches. The major ones are hatha yoga, raja yoga, bhakti yoga, karma yoga, jnana yoga and mantra yoga. One prepares the body and balances the prana or energy system with hatha yoga. Next the mind is explored and tamed with raja yoga. Karma yoga and bhakti yoga are powerful ways to purify and focus the mind and emotions. Mantra yoga purges the psyche or deeper levels of mind. Jnana yoga is direct enquiry into the self. Each type of yoga is complementary to the other types. An integral approach is more balanced, faster and safer. Yogic practices must be done regularly, sincerely, with faith and over a long time to obtain good results.

Awareness

Awareness of the present moment is the most important key in any type of yoga. Yogic practice done without awareness is not yogic practice at all. The practitioner is constantly required to be conscious of the experience generated at that moment and place. This training of being mindful of everything within and around allows us to understand the body and mind in relation to the environment. When something harmful and hurtful is happening, we receive the warning sign in time to stop the process. Similarly, when something beneficial is happening, we can appreciate it and encourage the process. We also start to understand how our mind is working. We observe our thoughts, considering where they come from (our desires, *iccha*) and how they influence our behaviour (action, *karma*). This initiates the process of learning about and improving the self.

The following is a list of some selected practices that are helpful to all, irrespective of the type of cancer. The list can be endless, so please do not think your practice should be limited to these practices. Some of these practices have been discussed already in chapter 5. The techniques for performing the remaining practices are described in the practice section at the end of this chapter, along with general as well as special precautions for cancer patients. Remember that one should choose, learn and practise them under the guidance of a qualified yoga teacher according to individual needs and capacities. It is not at all advisable to read a book and experiment on oneself or others.

The practices fall under the following headings. They are listed in order of learning; the sequence in daily practice is different. Mantras can be introduced at any suitable time during the learning process.

- Basic asanas
- Breath awareness
- Correct breathing (abdominal (diaphragmatic) and thoraco-abdominal breathing)
- Cleansing practices (shatkarmas)
- Balanced combination of asanas to suit individual needs
- Pranayama
- Yoga nidra
- Yamas and niyamas
- Dharana
- Bhakti yoga
- Karma yoga
- Mantra chanting and japa.

Basic asanas

One begins connecting with the body by practising some very simple asanas such as the pawanmuktasana part 1 series, tadasana (palm tree pose), tiryaka tadasana (swaying palm tree pose), kati chakrasana (waist rotating pose), marjari-asana (cat pose) and sphinx asana. The awareness should be inside the body where the movements are happening. These asanas are very gentle so almost everyone is able to do them, and they do not create any harmful effects. Practise them as much as you can comfortably manage. The quality of awareness is more important than the number of rounds or trying to achieve perfection.

These simple asanas are very powerful in releasing muscular stiffness and tension, improving the circulation of blood and prana and scavenging waste materials and toxins. To begin with they remove tamas and bring in rajas. The body will begin feeling lighter, more energetic and minor pains and discomforts will go away. The appetite and digestive ability will improve. Sleep patterns will stabilize. As one becomes adept, one synchronizes the breath with the physical movement under the guidance of the teacher and the awareness becomes meditative. At this stage, slowly sattwa starts to rise. The mood improves substantially and in spite of difficult situations a kind of pleasant, peaceful feeling is experienced internally. Self-confidence is restored. One starts understanding the needs of one's body.

Breath awareness

Next, one learns awareness of the breath. Simply observe each ingoing and outgoing natural, spontaneous breath closely. Do not alter the pattern of breathing. Watch how the breath enters the body, where it goes, how deep or shallow it is, how fast or slowly it flows, how it reverses its path and leaves the body, what sensations it creates as it flows in and out, what happens to the energy levels in the body as the breath flows in and out, what goes on inside the mind simultaneously as breath awareness continues, and so on.

164

This practice directs the normally extroverted mind to turn inward and become attentive to what is happening inside. It is a very easy and simple practice and at the same time very profound. It makes the mind quiet and brings it to a centre. The turmoil in the mind either stops or one is able to observe it with a neutral attitude and find a way out. If the mind is already calm and balanced, it sets it on course for its inner journey to find the higher self. At times many buried thoughts and emotions are brought to the surface. This simple practice gives us an opportunity to become aware of and deal with these unconscious memories appropriately. It is an effective tool with wide-ranging applications, from releasing normal day-to-day stress and managing various disease states to the highest spiritual quest.

Breath awareness can be practised by every age group, anywhere, by people of all levels of intellect, in all physical states and in most emotional states.

Correct breathing

Learning to breathe correctly is the next step. Deep quiet breathing, using the diaphragm and allowing the abdominal muscles to balloon out with inhalation and relax with exhalation is the correct way to breathe. This is known as abdominal breathing.

The breath sustains our life. We breathe in oxygen and prana and we breathe out waste material like carbon dioxide. Muscular effort is required in the breathing process. It costs us some calories and demands some oxygen. Diaphragmatic breathing, popularly known as abdominal breathing, is the most efficient way of breathing. It helps us acquire large amounts of oxygen with a minimum expenditure of energy. Here the main muscle used in respiration is the diaphragm. As it contracts and moves downward into the abdominal cavity, the lower areas of the lungs expand fully, the abdominal organs are pushed down and the abdomen balloons out. By the law of gravity the lower parts of the lungs receive a greater blood supply. In diaphragmatic breathing air enters these lower parts of the lungs, which optimizes the exchange of life-giving oxygen and waste carbon dioxide between the blood and the air.

In ordinary breathing, most people use the chest muscles predominantly, thus expanding and contracting the chest. This means that the incoming breath flows mainly to the upper area of the lungs, where the blood supply is not as great as it is in the lower lungs. There is a mismatch between the availability of blood and air. Extra breaths have to be taken to compensate for the mismatch, and the cost of breathing goes up.

As the abdominal muscles expand and contract rhythmically with breathing in and out, the mental stress stored in them in the form of increased muscle tone is released and the muscles relax. The mind calms down and energy levels improve. This creates a feeling of wellbeing. The rhythmic movement of the diaphragm gently massages the abdominal organs, improving their functioning.

Cleansing practices

The hatha yoga cleansing practices, popularly known as *shatkarmas* or *kriyas* must be learned and practised under expert supervision, assuming that the state of the body permits them to be practised. Jala neti, kunjal kriya and laghoo shankhaprakshalana (LSP) are strong and effective practices for cleansing the head and neck area, the chest and upper abdominal area and the abdominal and pelvic areas respectively.

These practices remove waste material at the physical level. They stimulate prana in the respective areas, thus indirectly removing harmful materials at even the cellular level. They purge the mind of thoughts, memories and emotions and throw out a lot of stored rubbish. The functioning of the respiratory and digestive systems is improved and the kidneys are flushed out. They relieve constipation, nausea and indigestion, purify the blood of waste materials, remove excess mucus from the respiratory

166

system, improve the appetite, remove fatigue and elevate depressed moods. *Asana Pranayama Mudra Bandha* is recommended for further reading.

Precaution: These practices are not recommended in low energy states, just after surgery, during or just after chemotherapy or radiotherapy and in selected cases of cancer affecting the head and neck area, respiratory and digestive organs.

Balanced asana program

According to the individual needs, one or two other asanas can be added to the basic asanas that have been described. The addition of a forward bending, a backward bending and a balancing asana help make a balanced asana program. It is suggested that you choose one of the following: saithalyasana, janu sirshasana, shashankasana or supta pawanmuktasana for forward bending; ardha shalabhasana, bhujangasana, kandharasana, ardha ushtrasana or saral dhanurasana for backward bending, and eka pada pranamasana, natarajasana or eka padasana from the balancing group. As a relaxation posture choose either shavasana, makarasana, advasana or matsya kridasana. For the practice of pranayama and dharana one of the following meditative asanas can be perfected: siddhasana/siddha yoni asana, ardha padmasana/padmasana, swastikasana or vajrasana. *Asana Pranayama Mudra Bandha* is recommended for further reading.

Pranayama

After initially preparing the body and mind with the basic asanas, breath awareness and cleansing practices, do the pre-pranayama and breath awareness practices. These involve learning to control the length and depth of the breath. After doing these practices, abdominal breathing, thoracic breathing and full yogic breathing may be learnt. Also learn to observe the duration of inhalation and exhalation, their inter-relationship and any changes in their proportion or ratio. Nadi shodhana pranayama, kapalbhati pranayama, bhramari pranayama and ujjayi pranayama are all very useful in our effort to manage cancer. *Asana Pranayama Mudra Bandha* is recommended for further reading.

The breath is a vehicle for prana. Through our breath we connect to the universal energy, cosmic prana or prakriti. We constantly derive energy from and send out our energy to the cosmos through the breath. All living beings link with each other and with the cosmos through their breath and thoughts. We often experience a rise in our energy level when we are in the presence of energetic people. The opposite is also equally true. In the presence of some people we feel drained of energy.

We generally have full voluntary control over our muscles and joints, but most of our internal organs are not under the control of our will. The breathing process is borderline in relation to conscious control; though it can function involuntarily, it can also be brought under voluntary control to a certain extent. The breath thus serves as a bridge between the body and mind, an area that we can control and an area beyond our control. The state of the mind and body can be manipulated by manipulating the breath. The yogic view is that the process of inhaling represents oxidation or catabolism or release of usable energy. It has a stimulating and awakening effect on the mind. The process of exhaling represents anabolism or storage of energy. It has a calming and introverting effect on the mind. Holding the breath stills the mind and allows it to become one-pointed. By modifying the pattern of breathing we can modify the physical, pranic and mental states. Various pranayama practices offer this possibility.

Precaution: Pranayama should be practised only according to the capacity of the individual. Never use any force or allow the lungs to undergo undue strain. Practise only under the guidance of a qualified teacher. People with high blood pressure or a heart problem should not practise inner or outer *kumbhaka,* retention of the breath, without the guidance of an expert.

Yoga nidra

The next practice is yoga nidra, a guided practice of relaxation and *pratyahara* (withdrawing the mind from external sense objects and directing it inward). An option in the practice is to also include *dharana* (concentrating the mind so that it becomes one-pointed and fixed on a single activity or object). Yoga nidra was first devised by Swami Satyananda Saraswati and made available to yoga practitioners in 1968.

In this practice the consciousness rests between the fully awake state and the sleep state. One is aware of one's dream state, but not of one's environment. One remains in a subconscious state. Yoga nidra can be given by a teacher or an audio recording may be used. Yoga nidra provides total physical, mental and emotional relaxation. Physical relaxation provides rest and the opportunity for the body to rejuvenate and heal. Mental relaxation allows mental conditionings and defences to be dropped. All expectations, logic and pre-conceived ideas are pushed aside and one enters into the state of one's natural self, releasing many self-created tensions. During yoga nidra, emotional relaxation allows suppressed emotions to float up into conscious awareness. Such emotions can be experienced from the position of a witness, enabling them to be understood from a different perspective and so dealt with objectively. This can put an end to stressful, emotionally charged situations of the past. Yoga nidra is a very powerful tool for combating stress of any kind and for the management of any disease, including cancer.

All types of tension lower the effectiveness of the immune system. When the immune response of the body is less than optimum, many enemies start raising their heads. Cancer is one such strong enemy that is difficult to keep in check. When we observe our internal mental environment and keep it reasonably clean by removing the negative tendencies and flooding it with positive attitudes and states, we boost our immune system and help prevent the seeds of cancer from germinating or growing. When the mind experiences negative states such as worry, depression, frustration, anger, jealousy

169

and revenge, the body's defence mechanisms are adversely affected and cancer has a greater chance of developing a foothold.

In the profound mental relaxation of yoga nidra, the artificial defence barriers put up by the mind drop, making the contents of the mind accessible for exploration and due action. We store much unwanted material, responsible for much of our distress, in the mind. The roots of cancer may be lying in this negative state of mind. The cancer may be feeding itself on this unwanted dross of the mind without our knowledge. The practice can also be used to explore and know what kind of thoughts and attitudes we harbour in the mind without being conscious of it. This gives us the chance to make changes as needed to improve our relationship with life. We can face the contents of our mind objectively, as a witness. Fears, anxieties and insecurities can be addressed without identifying and becoming involved with them, or coloured by them. We need to rid ourselves of this tamas which contaminates our natural sattwic state.

Yoga nidra can be specifically designed to enhance healing. For this purpose, the instructions guide the listener to tune into the cosmic energy. Then, through the vehicle of the breath this healing energy is drawn in and directed to a specific area.

Yoga nidra can also be used to utilize the power of our will. When a thought is wilfully planted in the subconscious mind, it always works its way to realization. During profound states of relaxation in the practice of yoga nidra, one can make contact with the subconscious mind. In this receptive mental state, the same resolve is repeatedly planted. The resolve is repeated twice during the practice of yoga nidra – just after the internalization process which induces physical relaxation in preparation for yoga nidra, and at the end of yoga nidra just before the process of externalization. In due time the resolve or thought becomes a reality. In this way the practice of yoga nidra can bring about a desired change in attitude and transform the personality totally. (*Yoga Nidra*, published by Yoga Publications Trust, is recommended for further reading.)

170

Yama and niyama

Before attempting dharana, or meditative practice, it is necessary to purify the mind by observing the yamas or self-restraints, and niyamas or personal disciplines, the first two steps of raja yoga. We have already discussed the yamas and niyamas earlier in this chapter.

First we learn to know our body, mind and prana through the practices of asana and breath awareness. This gives us some control over our body, mind and prana, and we can start to rectify their limitations by using asanas, the cleansing practices, pranayama and yoga nidra. Once tamas is reduced adequately, then rajas must be brought under control by purifying the mind through pranayama, yoga nidra, yama/niyama and dharana. When the mind has a lot of tamas, it is dull, lazy, disinterested, insecure and pessimistic. Under the influence of rajas, it wakes up, is active and interested, but lacks focus and direction. It jumps from one point to another like a mad monkey and gets nowhere. It is greedy, jealous, self-centred and lacks discrimination. The practice of yama/niyama and subsequently the practice of dharana train the mind to subdue rajas and enhance sattwa.

Dharana

The practice of dharana gives the mind a focus to attach itself to. As the mind, with focused awareness, becomes absorbed on the given focus rajas decreases and the original sattwa manifests, leading the practitioner into states of *dhyana*, undisturbed focused awareness. The original, untainted nature of the higher self is revealed; yoga or union takes place. Dharana practice trains one to connect with the atman, the inner source of life. One starts drawing on one's inner strength and becomes self-reliant. The cancer is burnt in the fire of the purity of sattwa.

The practices of dharana also train the mind to stay on one focus. A focused mind is a very powerful entity, like a focused ray of light or laser beam. It can overcome any obstacle and reach its goal. A sick person can easily become

171

preoccupied thinking about their health and lose their clarity of mind, decision-making ability and the willpower and self-confidence to implement decisions. Dharana practices lift a sick person out of a mood of depression and dejection and help one to regain the lost mental faculties of clarity, willpower, confidence and so on. One learns to take the reins of life back in one's hands.

A number of meditation practices are recommended. Ajapa japa, which focuses the attention on the breath and its sound is highly recommended. Another important practice is trataka, gazing at a *jyoti* or candle flame, or on the *ishta deva*, a personal symbol representing higher consciousness. A third equally powerful practice is mantra meditation. Yet another practice is antar mouna. Each practice has a different method of directing the mind. In ajapa japa it is by following the breath and its sound in a certain way, in trataka it is by concentrating on a visual symbol, in mantra meditation it is focusing on the sound, and in antar mouna on the thoughts.

Precautions: When first learning meditation a practitioner needs to be guided by a teacher. With experience one can use an audio recording. When one becomes adept, one can practise independently. Dharana practices may or may not work well with depressed and introverted people. People with a history of mental disorders should refrain from this practice.

Sure Ways to Self-Realization, Meditations from the Tantras and *Dharana Darshan*, published by Yoga Publications Trust, are recommended for further reading.

Bhakti yoga

The path of bhakti yoga can also be followed. Bhakti yoga purifies and stabilizes the mind effectively, and leads into a relationship with the Cosmic Self, which offers unfailing support. In bhakti yoga one channels the emotions in a particular direction without any expectation of personal gain. The object that the emotions are directed towards is called the *ishta*. Usually it is a personal god or guru, the spiritual master, but one can choose an act of service where the person served is seen as a representative of or a child of the ishta. There is a strong attraction for the ishta, the beloved one (or the activity), but no attachment or possessiveness. Initially an effort may be needed to redirect the emotions that are flowing in various directions and to strengthen the bond and establish a relationship with the ishta. The relationship with God is generally based on love, nurture, devotion, service, friendship or passion. The relationship is for one's entire lifetime, during which time the emotions may change and/or expand.

The ancient scriptures describe nine ways, known as *navadha bhakti*, of establishing and strengthening the relationship of the bhakta or devotee with the beloved. Basically this involves remembering, worshiping and serving the ishta or object of devotion in various ways. These include ritualistic worship, singing devotional songs, repeating the ishta's name, listening to stories of his glories, being in his presence, listening to his teachings and offering help in carrying out his work. These are some of the common practices for establishing bhakti. This approach mainly applies to a personal god or guru. It helps to develop trust and faith that the ishta will offer one support. The devotee feels inspired to develop the good qualities of the ishta. The ishta's spiritual teachings are also imbibed.

In *Ramacharitamanas*, nine methods of bhakti are described:
1. Satsang, being in the company of saints or people who are good and pure
2. Listening to the glorious stories of the Lord with interest
3. Serving the guru with humility
4. Singing the glory of the Lord with a simple heart
5. Mantra japa and worshipping the Lord with faith
6. Being of good character by developing control over the senses, detachment towards one's actions and fulfilling one's duties
7. Finding the Lord everywhere and in every being
8. Being content with whatever one gets and refraining from finding fault with others

9. Simplicity, abstaining from shrewdness, faith in the Lord and equanimity in opposing conditions, such as pleasure and pain.

Bhakti yoga provides inspiration, hope, assistance and the strength to meet the afflictions of life with courage. It can bear fruit quickly when a relationship is established with Him. In the present age, known as *kali yuga*, the main *sadhana*, or spiritual practice, is *kirtan* or singing the Lord's name together in a group.

Serving humanity with the idea that the Lord is residing in every being and that one is serving Him when serving humanity is also bhakti. Offering or dedicating all one's actions to Him, doing everything for Him is also bhakti. For example, while cooking one thinks "I am cooking for Him", while doing office work one thinks, "I am doing it to please Him", while taking a shower one thinks, "I should be at my best when I present myself to Him," and so on.

Upasana: In the Presence of the Divine and *Samarpan: Living the Divine Connection,* published by Yoga Publications Trust, are recommended for further reading.

Karma yoga

Karma yoga is yet another way to remove tamas from the body and mind. Karma yoga is the principal teaching of the *Bhagavad Gita*. *Karma* means action. A person cannot live without action. Through these activities, whether day-to-day or of major consequence, one can learn, grow and purify the mind. The process of converting ordinary routine actions into a tool for spiritual progress is karma yoga. The attitude behind an action is of paramount importance here. The activity itself strengthens rajas. The attitude of karma yoga behind the action will convert it to sattwa. If the attitude is not correct, then it can usher in rajas or tamas as well. In karma yoga there is an eagerness to work and there is a special attitude towards the work. Work is properly planned with a clear, achievable goal and a detailed method of execution. The goal should be as selfless as possible, or at least not harmful to anyone. When the actual work starts, the attention shifts from the result of the work to how best one can do it. The awareness is one-pointed on the process of working. The work is dedicated to the Lord or humanity. Whatever the ultimate outcome is one remains steady and balanced. If the outcome is good, one does not feel excessively elated, but remains aware of the Lord's grace and appreciates the assistance of others. If the outcome is not so good, one does not take it to heart, but finds a lesson to learn from it.

Mantra chanting and japa

Mantra chanting and mantra japa cleanse the subconscious and unconscious mind of *samskaras*, deeply imprinted past experiences. The instinct, dependent on the contents of the collective unconscious mind, can also be purified and refined with mantra. Only a guru, a highly evolved person, can guide us in mantra yoga. In mantra japa the selected mantra, usually of a few syllables, is repeated over and over using a *mala*, a string of 108 beads, either verbally, whispering or mentally; sometimes it is written down. In mantra chanting usually a longer composition of sounds is sung in a beautiful rhythm and tune. It can consist of a few to a few hundred verses. Faith and one-pointed awareness are important ingredients of the practice. One can use an appropriate picture of a deity, a yantra or the sound vibrations of the mantra itself to fix the awareness on. A *yantra* is a symmetrical geometrical figure, representing a certain concept in a symbolic way. Lighting a *deepak* or candle, incense, offering flowers or similar simple rituals can make the atmosphere conducive to the practice. Mantra japa and chanting can be practised lightly, five minutes to an hour or so every day, or as an *anushthana,* an extensive practice for several hours a day over many days in a retreat situation. There are certain rules to be followed while doing anushthana.

The repetitive sound vibrations of mantra produce a vibratory force that works subtly on the psyche and brings about a healing change. It awakens the person's inner strength to achieve the set goal. When the mind is focused with one aim, of restoring health, then that thought is charged with tremendous energy and fructifies into reality. Mantra chanting and prayers can work miracles in this manner.

The Mahamrityunjaya mantra is a specific healing mantra. It can be chanted by the individual or by family members or friends. See the practice section at the end of this chapter.

Fig. 7.3: Yogic Tools

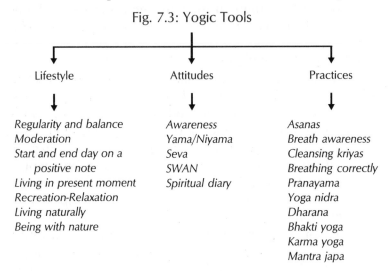

Lifestyle	Attitudes	Practices
Regularity and balance	Awareness	Asanas
Moderation	Yama/Niyama	Breath awareness
Start and end day on a	Seva	Cleansing kriyas
positive note	SWAN	Breathing correctly
Living in present moment	Spiritual diary	Pranayama
Recreation-Relaxation		Yoga nidra
Living naturally		Dharana
Being with nature		Bhakti yoga
		Karma yoga
		Mantra japa

Practices for individual cancers

Yoga is a holistic science and so its practices are not disease-specific. A balanced yoga program should serve the purpose. We do, however, recommend the practice of one asana that draws prana to the area, one pranayama to stimulate the prana in the affected area, and a purifying practice for the relevant *chakra* (subtle centre of concentrated energy in pranamaya kosha), called *chakra shuddhi*, in addition to a balanced program. Mantra chanting and a meditation of one's choice are highly recommended to complete the yoga program. Chakra shuddhi practices are beyond the scope of this book and readers are advised to contact a qualified, experienced teacher.

176

Table 7.1: Practices for Individual Cancers

Breast	*Gomukhasana, ujjayi pranayama, anahata shuddhi*
Cervix	*Bhadrasana and swastikasana, nadi shodhana pranayama, nasikagra drishti, mooladhara shuddhi*
Colon or kidney	*Swastikasana, nadi shodhana pranayama, swadhisthana shuddhi*
Prostate, ovary or uterus	*Swastikasana, nadi shodhana pranayama, swadhisthana shuddhi*
Stomach or liver	*Vajrasana, nadi shodhana pranayama, manipura shuddhi*
Lungs	*Gomukhasana, prana mudra, ujjayi pranayama, anahata shuddhi*
Oral cavity	*Bhramari pranayama, ajna shuddhi*
Throat	*Ujjayi pranayama, vishuddhi shuddhi*
Brain	*Bhramari pranayama, ajna shuddhi*
Blood	*Pawanmuktasana part 1 series, nadi shodhana pranayama, vishuddhi and ajna shuddhi*
Bone and muscles	*Pawanmuktasana part 1 series, ujjayi pranayama, mooladhara shuddhi*

177

MANTRA

Mantra chanting on waking in the morning

1. Mahamrityunjaya mantra: This mantra restores health at all levels. The Satyananda Yoga tradition recommends chanting of the Mahamrityunjaya mantra 11 times on waking first thing in the morning, even before getting out of bed. It is also recommended to aid recovery from an illness or from ill-fate. In this case it is usually chanted 108 times, either by oneself, a family member or by a well-wisher. It can also be chanted for the peace of a departed soul. The chanting can be done alone or in a group, once or every day. In Satyananda Yoga ashrams and centres and in the homes of devotees, it is chanted 108 times every Saturday evening for the wellbeing of everyone in this universe.

Technique

On waking in the morning, sit up comfortably while still in bed. Close the eyes. Become aware of the body and the breath. Then focus the awareness at the eyebrow centre, visualizing the symbol of a jyoti, a candle flame. Make a sankalpa, a resolve, for good health at all levels, physical, mental, emotional, social and spiritual. Start chanting the mantra with full conviction and clear pronunciation. At the end of 11 rounds chant 'Om shantih shantih shantih' once. Sit still for a few seconds.

ॐ त्र्यम्बकं यजामहे सुगन्धिं पुष्टिवर्धनम् ।
उर्वारुकमिव बन्धनात् मृत्योर्मुक्षीय मामृतात् ॥
ॐ शान्ति: शान्ति: शान्ति: ।

Om tryambakam yajaamahe sugandhim pushtivardhanam.
Urvaarukamiva bandhanaat mrityormuksheeya maamritaat.
Om shaantih shaantih shaantih.

2. Gayatri Mantra: This mantra sharpens the intellect and assists the dormant faculties of the mind to manifest, improving perception, analysis, creativity and decision-making. The Satyananda Yoga tradition recommends chanting this mantra 11 times immediately after chanting the Mahamrityunjaya mantra on waking. It is a useful spiritual practice for school students to chant Gayatri manta 108 times just after pranayama at or before sunrise. It can also be a mantra for personal spiritual practice.

Technique

After chanting the Mahamrityunjaya mantra on waking in the morning, and maintaining awareness of the flame at the eyebrow centre, make a sankalpa, a resolve for accurate perception, clear thinking and wisdom. Then chant the Gayatri mantra 11 times followed again by 'Om shantih, shantih, shantih'. Sit still for few seconds.

ॐ भूर्भुव: सुव: तत्सवितुर्वरेण्यं ।
भर्गो देवस्य धीमहि धियो यो न: प्रचोदयात् ॥
ॐ शान्ति: शान्ति: शान्ति: ।

Om bhoorbhuvah svah tatsaviturvarenyam.
Bhargo devasya dheemahi dhiyo yo nah prachodayaat.
Om shaantih shaantih shaantih.

3. 32 Names of Durga: This mantra removes obstacles from one's life. It gives one the inner strength and wisdom to overcome any obstacle that life presents. The Satyananda Yoga tradition recommends chanting of this mantra 3 times immediately after chanting the Mahamrityunjaya and Gayatri mantras on waking. It can be used more often during the day in times of difficulties. It can also be a part of an anushthana or intensive chanting done on special occasions such as Navaratri.

Technique

Maintaining awareness on the flame at the eyebrow centre after chanting the Mahamrityunjaya and Gayatri mantras, make a sankalpa, a resolve, to overcome all obstacles in life and chant the 32 names of Durga (*Durgadvatrimshannama-mala*) 3 times. End with 'Om shantih, shantih, shantih'.

ॐ दुर्गा दुर्गार्तिशमनी दुर्गापद्विनिवारिणी ।
दुर्गमच्छेदिनी दुर्गसाधिनी दुर्गनाशिनी ॥
दुर्गतोद्धारिणी दुर्गनिहन्त्री दुर्गमापहा ।
दुर्गमज्ञानदा दुर्गं दैत्यलोकदवानला ॥
दुर्गमा दुर्गमालोका दुर्गमात्मस्वरूपिणी ।
दुर्गमार्गप्रदा दुर्गमविद्या दुर्गमाश्रिता ॥
दुर्गमज्ञानसंस्थाना दुर्गमध्यानभासिनी ।
दुर्गमोहा दुर्गमगा दुर्गमार्थस्वरूपिणी ॥
दुर्गमासुरसंहन्त्री दुर्गमायुधधारिणी ।
दुर्गमांगी दुर्गमता दुर्गम्या दुर्गमेश्वरी ॥
दुर्गभीमा दुर्गभामा दुर्गभा दुर्गदारिणी ।
ॐ शान्तिः शान्तिः शान्तिः ॥

Om durgaa durgaartishamanee durgaapadvinivaarinee.
Durgamachchhedinee durgasaadhinee durganaashinee.
Durgatoddhaarinee durganihantree durgamaapahaa.
Durgamajnaanadaa durga daityalokadavaanalaa.
Durgamaa durgamaalokaa durgamaatmasvaroopinee.
Durgamaargapradaa durgamavidyaa durgamaashritaa.
Durgamajnaanasamsthaanaa durgamadhyaanabhaasinee.
Durgamohaa durgamagaa durgamaarthasvaroopinee.
Durgamaasurasamhantree durgamaayudhadhaarinee.
Durgamaangee durgamataa durgamyaa durgameshvaree.
Durgabheemaa durgabhaamaa durgabhaa durgadaarinee.
Om shaantih shaantih shaantih.

Shanti mantras from the Upanishads

Shanti mantras invoke *shanti*, meaning peace, or in a broader sense, goodwill. Many mantras can be included in this category. They are like prayers for good wishes. Three of the most commonly used Shanti mantras in the Satyananda Yoga tradition are given below. The first one is usually chanted before starting a task, and the other two at the end of a task or activity. The last one can also be used as a prayer.

1. ॐ सह नाववतु। सह नौ भुनक्तु। सह वीर्यं करवावहै।
   तेजस्विनावधीतमस्तु। मा विद्विषावहै।
   ॐ शान्ति: शान्ति: शान्ति: ॥

   Om saha naavavatu. Saha nau bhunaktu. Saha veeryam karavaavahai.
   Tejasvinaavadheetamastu. Maa vidvishaavahai.
   Om shaantih shaantih shaantih.

   Om. May the Lord protect both teacher and disciple, may He nourish us both and may we work together with full energy.
   Let our learning be full of brilliance. Let us not have ill-will for each other.
   Om peace, peace, peace.

2. ॐ पूर्णमद: पूर्णमिदं पूर्णात् पूर्णमुदच्यते।
   पूर्णस्य पूर्णमादाय पूर्णमेवावशिष्यते।
   ॐ शान्ति: शान्ति: शान्ति: ॥

   Om poornamadah poornamidam poornaat poornamudachyate.
   Poornasya poornamaadaaya poornamevaavashishyate.
   Om shaantih shaantih shaantih.

   That is full, this is full. From fullness, fullness has come.
   If the fullness is removed, only fullness remains.
   Om peace, peace, peace.

3. असतो मा सद्गमय। तमसो मा ज्योतिर्गमय। मृत्योर्माऽमृतं गमय।
सर्वेषां स्वस्तिर्भवतु। सर्वेषां शान्तिर्भवतु। सर्वेषां पूर्णं भवतु। सर्वेषां
मंगलं भवतु।
लोका: समस्ता: सुखिनो भवन्तु।
ॐ त्र्यम्बकं यजामहे सुगन्धिं पुष्टिवर्धनम् ।
उर्वारुकमिव बन्धनात् मृत्योर्मुक्षीय मामृतात् ॥
ॐ शान्ति: शान्ति: शान्ति:।

त्वमेव माता च पिता त्वमेव
त्वमेव बन्धुश्च सखा त्वमेव ।
त्वमेव विद्या द्रविणं त्वमेव
त्वमेव सर्वं मम देव देव ॥
हरि ॐ ।

Asato maa sadgamaya. Tamaso maa jyotirgamaya.
Mrityormaa'mritam gamaya.
Sarveshaam svastirbhavatu. Sarveshaam shaantirbhavatu.
Sarveshaam poornam bhavatu. Sarveshaam mangalam
bhavatu.
Lokaah samastaah sukhino bhavantu.
Om tryambakam yajaamahe sugandhim pushtivardhanam.
Urvaarukamiva bandhanaat mrityormuksheeya maamritaat.
Om shaantih shaantih shaantih.

Tvameva maataa cha pitaa tvameva, tvameva bandhushcha
sakhaa tvameva.
Tvameva vidyaa dravinam tvameva, tvameva sarvam mama
deva deva.
Tvameva sarvam mama deva deva, tvameva sarvam mama
deva deva.
Hari Om.

From unreality lead me to reality! From ignorance to
enlightenment! From mortality to immortality!
May good befall all! May peace be unto all! May all attain
perfection! May all attain auspiciousness!
May all worlds be happy!

Mahamrityunjaya mantra for the health, happiness and prosperity of all.
Om peace, peace, peace.

Only You are my mother and my father.
Only You are my brother and my friend.
Only You are my knowledge (the power of understanding) and my wealth (of all kinds). O Lord of Lords!
You and only you are everything that I have.
Hari Om.

YAMA AND NIYAMA

Yama is the first step on the eightfold ladder of Patanjali's ashtanga yoga. It is the preliminary practice in every method of self-evolution, being the basic building block for *manava dharma*, the duties of human beings. At the same time, perfecting the yamas is not so easy. According to the raja yoga system there are five yamas:
1. *Ahimsa* (non-violence)
2. *Satya* (truthfulness)
3. *Asteya* (non-stealing)
4. *Brahmacharya* (control over the sensory organs)
5. *Aparigraha* (non-possessiveness).

Niyama is the second step on the ladder. The yamas and niyamas are loosely translated as 'self-restraints or social code of conduct', and 'personal observances or disciplines' respectively. The yamas help to harmonize the social environment and the niyamas help to harmonize the inner environment and transform the personality and attitudes. Both the yamas and niyamas prepare one for meditation practices. Every spiritual system has its own codes of conduct and personal observances. According to the raja yoga system there are five niyamas:
1. *Shaucha* (cleanliness)
2. *Santosha* (contentment)
3. *Tapas* (austerity)

4. *Swadhyaya* (self-study)
5. *Ishwara pranidhana* (surrender to the higher will or God).

As a first step on the spiritual journey, it is best to choose just one yama and one niyama and try to perfect them over a period of time. Choose any one of them – starting with the quality you feel most attracted to will make the task easier. During this time the remaining yamas and niyamas will automatically start flowering in your personality. You will find that you also grow stronger internally.

Ahimsa: *Himsa,* or violence, can be of three types: committed by the person himself; enacted through someone else; and approving of violence done by someone else. In any act of violence the motive is more important than the act itself. Violence can occur in action, in speech and in thoughts. Hence ahimsa (non-violence) should be observed not only in action, but also in speech and thoughts. A violent thinking pattern leads to violence in speech and action, so it is more important to observe ahimsa in the thoughts.

Ahimsa comes from strength and fearlessness, never from cowardice or weakness. Ahimsa is not a forced attitude; it spontaneously arises from the love, care and consideration felt for others and from a willingness to cooperate. Violence is born of attachment and desire. Violence is a reaction when a desire or attachment is not fulfilled. Developing non-attachment leads to a non-reactive nature and to ahimsa.

The attitude of seeing one's own self in every other living being leads to perfect ahimsa. In Swami Sivananda's words, "Ahimsa is cosmic love." It is essential to include yourself in the application and practice of ahimsa. Be non-violent to yourself.

Satya or truthfulness has various levels:
1. Truthfulness in speech.
2. Complete truthfulness, i.e. abstaining from hiding the truth or telling a half-truth, modifying the truth or colouring the truth with personal opinions.
3. Truthfully connecting one's beliefs, thoughts, speech and actions. This means speaking one's mind and doing what

184

is spoken or what is believed. In satya, there is no discrepancy between the three.

4. Speaking the truth and acting in accordance with the truth at the right time and in the right manner (without hurting anyone).
5. Truth can have many facets. What one knows and believes can be one part of the total truth. Another person's opinion can also be true, or the other part of the total truth. One who tries to know and accept this, so widening the concept of truth, has the attitude of a *satyagrahi*.
6. *Satyagraha* is insisting on and sticking to the truth in difficult and trying situations.

Asteya means not stealing someone else's belongings, including non-material possessions, not stealing someone else's ideas or words and presenting them as one's own. It means not stealing someone else's opportunity by using unfair means. The motive is more important than the act. This yama means being totally honest. Consuming more than one's needs can also mean stealing at times.

Brahmacharya, in its limited aspect, means celibacy. In a broader and more appropriate sense, it means reducing sense enjoyments to the extent that the mind can remain established in spiritual pursuits or can evolve itself.

There are three stages: *indriya sanyam,* exercising restraint over the senses, *indriya nigraha,* sense withdrawal, and *indriya jaya,* mastery over the senses. The type of food we eat, fasting, the company and associations we keep, adequate and appropriate physical activity, reading inspiring literature, associating with saintly people and exposure to sensual, tempting environments are important factors which influence this practice. Like the other yamas, brahmacharya needs to be observed in thought as well as in action. Some yogic practices assist in observing celibacy.

Aparigraha means possessing only the bare minimum. *Parigraha*, the desire to possess more, is the root cause of failure in all five yamas. This tendency in us comes from the instinct of self-preservation and the need to feel secure.

Aparigraha can be external and material, or internal and subtle. It arises from non-attachment and non-motivation.

Shaucha means cleanliness. The term is generally used for personal hygiene and cleanliness of the surroundings or external cleanliness. In cleanliness there is neatness and orderliness, which leads to efficiency. External cleanliness kindles the process of internal purification, purification of the mind. Positive forces in the cosmos are attracted to a clean place and a clean person.

Santosha is being happily content with whatever one has and in whatever situation one is placed in. It is never a passive quality. Generally, only when we know we have tried our hardest and made our best effort can we be content whatever the outcome may be. There needs to be spontaneous (not forced) acceptance and trust in a higher force to successfully practise santosha.

Tapas means a vow of austerity. It reflects self-control and the ability to tolerate any physical condition. Tapas can be external and physical, or internal and mental. It strengthens and purifies the body and mind, and accelerates spiritual growth. Austerities can be done either for the fulfilment of a specific desire or without any desire. Tapas is not physical or mental torture, but a practice to gradually increase endurance.

Swadhyaya is self-study, observing and analyzing oneself. *Swa* means 'self' and *adhyayana* means 'study'. It also means studying and learning by oneself, usually in the context of studying the scriptures. It is essential for the process of transformation and spiritual growth.

Ishwara pranidhana, surrender to the Divine or God, means having total faith in that higher reality and accepting everything that happens as God's wish. Living in this way is believing that whatever God decides is best for everyone concerned. No situation or event is rejected or condemned. Instead, we try to discover the lesson behind adversity. When things go well and we have favourable experiences, the credit also goes to God (the idea of non-doership). Surrender to God is expressed in thought, feeling and action.

Practical suggestions

- Take time to decide which yama and niyama to follow.
- Try to choose a yama and a niyama which seems closest to your nature and which feels most important to you.
- Observe this yama first in your behaviour and speech, and then gradually in your thoughts also.
- Try to observe the niyama in your outward behaviour as well as in your thoughts, beliefs and feelings.
- Start slowly. Be gentle but very firm with yourself. Be totally sincere.
- Remind yourself of the chosen yama and niyama at fixed times of the day; for example, on waking, after spiritual practice, before meals, when stepping out of the house and before going to bed.
- Remember the yama and niyama periodically during the day in the midst of any activity. Modify your actions and thoughts accordingly.
- Keep written reminders of the yama and niyama in prominent places around you; for example, on the work desk, next to the bed, on the dressing table mirror.
- Read stories about great people's views and experiments with life. This will inspire you as well as giving direction and support to your efforts.
- Be vigilant and regular in self-observation and self-analysis.
- Observe and analyze achievements and failures, the effects of rewards and punishments.
- Experiment with the various influencing factors and observe the effects.
- Writing a spiritual diary is useful.
- It might help to work out a method of self-assessment on a scale of 1 to 10. Before you start observing the yama and niyama, determine where you are on the scale. Then chart your progress.
- Discuss your progress periodically with an experienced person if possible.
- Remain humble. Avoid arrogance as you progress in this spiritual practice.

There will be times during the day when awareness of your yama-niyama will arise strongly and spontaneously and guide your behaviour. Try to also consciously and repeatedly bring in awareness of the yama and niyama during the day's activities and then evaluate the activity in the context of the yama and niyama. At the end of the day, analyze and evaluate your actions and reactions in the light of the yama and niyama.

Understanding, awareness, persistent effort and self-analysis are the four pillars to success in any spiritual practice. Do not lose heart when you do not succeed. Continue your efforts with fresh zeal and determination.

EIGHTEEN ITIES

A tool similar to the yamas and niyamas, but much subtler, is recommended by Swami Sivananda Saraswati of Rishikesh. It is known as the song of eighteen 'ities'.

Song of Eighteen 'Ities'
Serenity, Regularity, Absence of Vanity,
Sincerity, Simplicity, Veracity,
Equanimity, Fixity, Non-Irritability,
Adaptability, Humility, Tenacity,
Integrity, Nobility, Magnanimity,
Charity, Generosity, Purity.
Practise daily these eighteen 'ities',
You will soon attain immortality.

Try to cultivate one 'ity' at a time, for a certain length of time, such as one month, and then go on to the next one until all the 'ities' are covered. You can then repeat the cycle or choose some of the 'ities' to work on for a longer duration. You can choose either the 'ities' or the yamas and niyamas. The suggested method of practising the yamas and niyamas can also be applied to the eighteen 'ities'.

188

SWAN PRACTICE

SWAN is an acronym for Strength, Weakness, Ambition and Need. It is a self-analytical practice in which these four areas of the personality are observed and evaluated. As with the yamas and niyamas, the spiritual diary or the eighteen 'ities', the SWAN practice needs to be done with sincerity, honesty and gentleness in a non-judgemental way that is forgiving to oneself and also persistent. The practical suggestions given for the yamas and niyamas are also recommended to assist in the SWAN practice.

Stage 1: Observe yourself in order to identify your strengths or positive qualities, your weaknesses, limitations or negative qualities, your ambitions (desires you would like to attain but are not essential), and your needs (requirements necessary for your wellbeing). Continue making your observations for a few weeks and then shortlist the collected information. It is necessary to spend adequate time on this stage. Most of us feel that we know ourselves, but this is not really so. If we are in a hurry to go on to the second stage, we will miss many hidden aspect of ourselves.

Stage 2: Identify your current aim in life. Decide which strengths are useful and which weaknesses obstruct your aim. Decide which ambitions and needs should become your priority and which can wait. Make a daily note of your SWA and N as it shows up in your thoughts, feelings and behaviour that day. Note the changing pattern of your SWAN on a daily basis. Sometimes the strength manifests as a weakness in a certain context and a weakness may even become a strength in a particular scenario. Choose a strength that you would like to further strengthen and a weakness that you would like to overcome.

Stage 3: Employ one or more of the following methods to bring about the necessary change.

1. *Awareness*: In this practice you simply observe your thoughts, feelings and actions. The desired change automatically happens. No conflict or guilt is experienced.

189

2. *Drashta bhava* is observing with the attitude of a witness (as if you are watching a film). In this state of mind, it is as if you are two. One 'you' is the doer, which is thinking, feeling or acting, while the other 'you', the observer or *drashta*, is passively watching or witnessing the first 'you' doing the action without becoming involved in the event. The witnessing attitude is a more refined form of simple awareness.

3. *Manan*, contemplation or logical thinking. Choose a personality trait in yourself and contemplate the benefits and hazards it has had on your life and their future possibilities. When your mind is convinced, it will retain or discard the quality effortlessly. The study of biographies of inspiring people can be very supportive in this process, as it is demonstrated in their lives. Satsang or associating with good people and spending time with saints inspires us and helps us to imbibe the good qualities that are so strong in them.

4. *Pratipaksha bhava*, developing the opposite attitude. Rather than trying to remove the weaknesses, it may be more effective to work at increasing the strengths. When one is working on removing weaknesses, feelings such as frustration (due to lack of success) and guilt (due to perceived inadequacy) may become overpowering. In spite of all one's good-hearted attempts the negativity may keep coming with renewed force and zeal. It is much easier and safer to develop a positive quality than to rid oneself of a negative quality. In pratipaksha bhava one tries to cultivate an opposite positive attitude instead of trying to remove a negative attitude. For example, to reduce anger one can work at developing patience, tolerance, acceptance, feelings of brotherhood, compassion or love. Sage Patanjali says in the *Yoga Sutras* (2:33), "When the mind is disturbed by passions, one should practise pondering over their opposites."

5. *Sankalpa* means resolve or affirmation. When a sankalpa is made, we are using our willpower to accomplish

something. Sankalpa is a short affirmative sentence in the present tense repeated mentally three times at the beginning and end of yoga nidra with the full conviction that it will materialize. It is made with the faith that this resolve never fails. The sankalpa can also be repeated mentally at the end of meditation practice, as a prayer, on waking in the morning, just before going to bed or before a meal. Whenever repeating it, do so with full faith. For example, to overcome anger, the sankalpa can be 'I win over anger' or 'I am in full control of myself' or 'I think twice before speaking or acting' or 'I am balanced in all situations'. This does not mean that once a sankalpa is made one stops making any effort at self-transformation. A sankalpa provides us with inner strength and boosts our efforts.

SWAN practice in a nutshell

Set a fixed time, preferably at bedtime, to review the day's happenings and the associated thoughts, feelings and reactions. Try to limit the time to five to ten minutes. Maintain a spiritual diary, noting the following points very briefly and ensuring they are to the point. See the guidelines in the section on 'spiritual diary' below.

Stage 1: Preferably spend two to four weeks on this stage.
• Identify the **S**trengths, **W**eaknesses, **A**mbitions and **N**eeds.
• Shortlist the collected information.

Stage 2: Spend two weeks or more at this stage, until you are clear in your mind. Then add stage 3.
• Decide the priority amongst all the ambitions and needs.
• Identify the current aim(s) of life, depending on the ambitions and needs.
• Which strengths are necessary and which weaknesses are obstructive to the fulfilment of this aim?
• Identify the strengths, weaknesses, ambitions and needs that show up prominently each day.
• Which strength needs to be strengthened and which weakness needs to be overcome?

191

- What are the priorities for the ambitions and needs?

Stage 3: Continue to practise along with stage 2 as long as you need to.

- Gradually and gently bring about the necessary changes in your strengths and weaknesses using one or more of the following methods. Remember to be patient and non-judgemental and at the same time sincere and firm with yourself.

    1. Awareness
    2. Witnessing attitude
    3. Contemplation
    4. Developing the opposite quality
    5. Resolve.

SPIRITUAL DIARY

The practice of writing a diary is one of self-observation and self-analysis. It helps us to understand the workings of our mind, emotional make-up and behaviour patterns. It helps us connect with our inner self. Therefore, it is called a spiritual diary. One may also choose to keep a diary for other purposes, such as monitoring the course of the disease and one's health. We will restrict our discussion to the spiritual diary. Initially the diary needs to actually be written down, but later it can be gone through mentally.

Initially it is only a practice of self-observation. Maintain a passive witnessing attitude and avoid being judgemental at any cost. This process alone can produce the needed changes. Certain trends will emerge from these observations. After two or three months of passive observation, start analyzing the thoughts, emotions and behaviour responses to various stimuli. Be impartial and honest. Be gentle and patient with yourself. Identify the factors that trigger a particular thought, emotion or behaviour pattern. Identify the real causes behind them. Find and execute methods of transformation. Discuss with your guide or an experienced person. Periodically note the changes in your personality.

It is preferable to write the spiritual diary in a set format rather than in a free flowing style. It is less time consuming, facilitates clear thinking, important points are not missed out and it is easy to refer to in the future. Decide the format according to your needs and modify it periodically as needed. Let the format be light, short, clear and easy to respond to, while at the same time being appropriate. Give answer options that can simply be ticked. Alternatively, formulate questions in such a way that one word answers are possible.

Guidelines for writing a spiritual diary

Set aside a time for diary writing. Just before bedtime, review the day, make the entries in your diary, practise mantra japa and the meditation of your choice, and then go to bed.

Broadly speaking, a spiritual diary should cover the following areas:

1. *Lifestyle – regularity and balance*: Give a reason in one word for any lapse in relation to this aspect of lifestyle.
2. *Events during the day which created an impact*: Describe the thoughts, emotions and behaviour surrounding any such event, using just one word for each.
3. *The day in respect of the aim of life*: Facilitating/no impact/contrary/can't say. Give a reason in one word where appropriate.
4. *The day in respect of your yama and niyama*: Well observed/slipped out of mind/neglected knowingly/found difficult to bring into practice. Give the reason in one word where appropriate and if needed, suggest a possible remedy.
   Periodically evaluate how the yama and niyama are influencing your personality and your interactions with other people, and how you can improve your practice of yama and niyama.
5. *The day in the light of your SWAN*: Which SWAN came to the surface today?
   Periodically evaluate which measures can be taken to modify your SWAN and how successfully you are able to carry them out.

6. *Learning of the day*: Recognize this and briefly note it.
7. *Prayer of the day*:
   Healing the area of trauma
   Strength to overcome limitations
   Love for yourself and everyone.

ASANAS

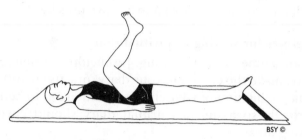

BSY ©

Pada Sanchalanasana (cycling)

Stage 1: Lie down flat on the back with the legs together and straight. The arms should be by the sides, palms down, and the head, neck and spine in a straight line. Let the body relax.

Raise the right leg.

Bend the knee and bring the thigh to the chest.

Raise and straighten the leg completely. Then lower the straight leg in a forward movement.

Bend the knee and bring it back to the chest to complete the cycling movement.

The heel should not touch the floor during the movement. Practise 10 times in a forward direction and then 10 times in reverse. Repeat with the left leg.

Breathing: Inhale while straightening the leg.

Exhale while bending the knee and bringing the thigh to the chest.

Stage 2: Raise both legs. Practise alternate cycling movements as though peddling a bicycle.

Practise 10 times forward and then 10 times backward.

Breathing: Breathe normally throughout.

Awareness: On the smoothness of the movement and proper coordination, especially while reverse cycling. When relaxing, be aware of the abdomen, hips, thighs and lower back, and the breath.

Contra-indications: Not to be performed by persons suffering from uncontrolled high blood pressure or high blood pressure with complications, or serious back conditions such as sciatica and slipped disc.

Benefits: Good for hip and knee joints. Strengthens abdominal and lower back muscles. Improves circulation. Improves digestion by stimulating prana in the abdominal area.

For cancer patients: It is contra-indicated in the presence of abdominal pain and for at least six weeks after abdominal surgery. It improves circulation and prevents deep vein thrombosis in the post-surgery period and in immobilized persons. It removes lethargy and elevates mood by mobilizing prana.

Practice note: Keep the rest of the body, including the head, flat on the floor throughout the practice. After completing each stage remain in the base position and relax until the respiration returns to normal. If cramping is experienced in the abdominal muscles, inhale deeply, gently pushing out the abdomen, and then relax the whole body with exhalation. Do not strain.

Supta Pawanmuktasana (leg lock pose)

Stage I: Lie down flat on the back with the legs together and straight. The arms should be by the sides, palms down, and the head, neck and spine in a straight line. Let the body relax.

Bend the right knee and bring the thigh to the chest.

Interlock the fingers and clasp the hands on the shin just below the right knee.

Keep the left leg straight and on the ground.

Inhale deeply, filling the lungs as much as possible.

Exhaling, raise the head and shoulders off the ground and without straining bring the right knee to the nose.

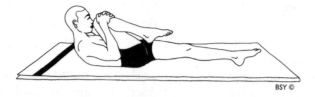

Remain in the final position for a few seconds.

While slowly inhaling, return to the base position.

Relax the body.

Repeat 3 times with the right leg and then 3 times with the left leg.

Practice note: Ensure that the straight leg remains in contact with the ground.

It is important to start with the right leg because it presses the ascending colon directly.

Follow with the left leg which presses the descending colon directly.

Stage 2: Remain in the starting position.

Bend both knees and bring the thighs to the chest.

Interlock the fingers and clasp the hands on the shin bones just below the knees.

Inhale deeply.

Exhaling, raise the head and shoulders and try to place the nose in the space between the two knees.

Hold the raised position for a few seconds, counting mentally.

Slowly lower the head, shoulders and legs while inhaling. Practise this 3 times.

Awareness: On the movement, the abdominal pressure, and the breath.

Contra-indications: Not to be performed by persons suffering from high blood pressure or serious back conditions such as sciatica and slipped disc without expert guidance.

Benefits: Supta pawanmuktasana strengthens the lower back muscles and loosens the spinal vertebrae. It massages the

196

abdomen and the digestive organs and is therefore very effective in removing wind and constipation. By massaging the pelvic muscles and reproductive organs, it is also useful for menstrual problems.

For cancer patients: It is not to be performed by persons with advanced cancer of any of the abdominal organs.

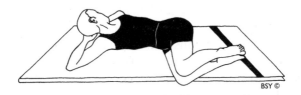

Supta Udarakarshanasana (sleeping abdominal stretch pose)

Lie down flat on the back with the legs together and straight. The arms should be by the sides, palms down, and the head, neck and spine in a straight line. Let the body relax.

Bend the knees and place the soles of both feet flat on the floor, directly in front of the buttocks.

Keep the knees and feet together throughout the practice. Interlock the fingers of both hands, place the palms under the back of the head and let the elbows touch the floor.

Breathe in, and while breathing out, slowly lower the legs to the right, trying to bring the knees down to the floor. The feet should remain in contact with each other, although the left foot will move slightly off the floor. At the same time, gently turn the head and neck in the opposite direction to the legs. This will give a uniform twisting stretch to the entire spine. Hold the breath in the final position while mentally counting three seconds.

While breathing in, raise both legs to the upright position. Keep the shoulders and elbows on the floor throughout.

Repeat on the left side to complete one round.

Practise 5 complete rounds.

Variation: Bend the knees and bring the thighs up to the chest. Interlock the fingers and place them behind the

197

head. Roll the body from side to side, keeping the elbows on the floor.

Breathing: Exhale while lowering the legs to the sides.

Hold the breath in the final position.

Inhale while raising the legs.

Awareness: On the twisting stretch of the paraspinal and abdominal muscles, and the breath.

Benefits: This asana gives an excellent stretch to the abdominal muscles and organs, and thereby helps to improve digestion and eliminate constipation. The twisting stretch of the spinal muscles relieves the strain and stiffness, especially in the lower back, caused by prolonged sitting. The pelvic and abdominal organs are toned through its massaging action.

Practice note: The distance of the feet from the buttocks determines the placement of the spinal twist. If the feet are about 60 cm from the buttocks, the adjustment is in the lower area of the spine. As the feet approach the buttocks, the adjustment rises up the spine. When the feet are next to the buttocks, the adjustment is in the area of the cardiac plexus. Therefore, moving the feet about 3 cm closer to the buttocks for each round works on each vertebra, bringing suppleness to the whole spinal column.

Sequence: This asana should be performed after forward and backward bending asanas or those that are strenuous on the lower back, and after sitting in chairs or in meditation asanas for extended periods of time. It is also performed after yoga nidra practice to reactivate relaxed muscles.

Rajju Karshanasana (pulling the rope)

Sit on the floor with the legs straight and together.

Keep the eyes open.

Imagine that there is a rope hanging in front of the body.

Breathe in while reaching up with the right hand as though to grasp the rope at a higher point.

Keep the elbow straight.

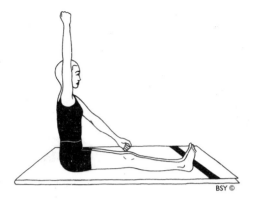

Look upward.

While breathing out, slowly pull the right arm down, putting power into it as though pulling the rope downwards. Let the eyes follow the downward movement of the hand.

Repeat with the left hand and arm to complete the first round.

Both arms do not move at the same time.

Practise 10 rounds.

Breathing: Inhale while raising the arm.

Exhale while lowering the arm.

Awareness: On the movement and stretch of the upper back and shoulder muscles, and the breath.

Benefits: This asana loosens the shoulder joints and stretches the upper back muscles. It firms the breast and develops the muscles of the chest.

For cancer patients: It is specially recommended after surgery for breast cancer.

Shashankasana (pose of the moon or hare pose)

Sit in vajrasana, placing the palms on the thighs just above the knees.

Close the eyes and relax, keeping the spine and head straight.

While inhaling, raise the arms above the head, keeping them straight and shoulder-width apart.

199

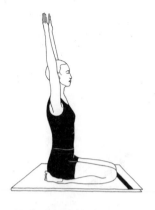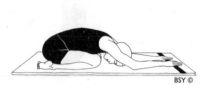

Exhale while bending the trunk forward from the hips. Keep the arms and head straight and in line with the trunk.

At the end of the movement, the hands and forehead should rest on the floor in front of the knees.

If possible, the arms and forehead should touch the floor at the same time.

Bend the arms slightly so that they are fully relaxed and let the elbows rest on the floor.

Retain the breath for up to 5 seconds in the final position. Then simultaneously inhale and slowly raise the arms and trunk to the vertical position. Keep the arms and head in line with the trunk.

Breathe out while lowering the hands to the knees.

This is one round.

Practise 3 to 5 rounds.

Duration: Beginners should slowly increase the length of time in the final position until they are able to hold it comfortably for at least 3 minutes with normal breathing. Those who wish to calm anger and frayed nerves should further increase the time to 10 minutes, breathing normally.

Awareness: Physical – in the final position, on the pressure of the abdomen against the thighs; on the alignment of arms, neck and head moving into and out of the asana; on the breath synchronized with the physical movement.

Spiritual – on manipura or swadhisthana chakra in the final position.

Contra-indications: Not to be performed by people with very high blood pressure, slipped disc or those who suffer from vertigo.

Benefits: This asana stretches and strengthens the back muscles and separates the individual vertebrae from each other, releasing pressure on the discs. Often nerve connections emanating from the spinal cord are squeezed by these discs, giving rise to various forms of backache.

This posture helps to relieve this problem in some cases and encourages the discs to resume their correct position. It also regulates the functioning of the adrenal glands. It tones the pelvic muscles and the sciatic nerves and is beneficial for both the male and female reproductive organs. Regular practice relieves constipation.

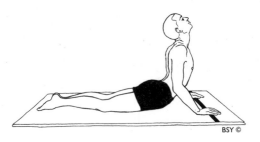

Bhujangasana (cobra pose)

Lie flat on the stomach with the legs straight, feet together and the soles of the feet uppermost.

Place the palms of the hands flat on the floor, below and slightly to the side of the shoulders, with the fingers together and pointing forward.

Position the arms so that the elbows point backward and are close to the sides of the body.

Rest the forehead on the floor and close the eyes.

Relax the whole body, especially the lower back.

Slowly raise the head.

Gently tilt the head backward, so that the chin points forward and the back of the neck is compressed, then raise the neck and finally the shoulders.

Straighten the elbows, using the back muscles first, then the arm muscles to raise the trunk further and arch the back.

In the final position, the pubic bone remains in contact with the floor and the navel is raised a maximum of 3 cm. If the navel is raised too high, the bend tends to be in the knees and not in the back.

The arms may or may not be straight; this will depend on the flexibility of the back.

Hold the final position.

To return to the starting position, slowly release the upper back by bending the arms, lowering the navel, chest, shoulders and finally the forehead to the floor.

Relax the lower back muscles.

This is one round.

Breathing: Inhale while raising the torso.

Breathe normally in the final position or retain the breath if the pose is held for a short time.

Exhale while lowering the torso.

Duration: Practise up to 5 rounds, gradually increasing the length of time in the final position.

Awareness: Physical – on the smooth, systematic arching movement of the back, the stretching of the abdomen, and on synchronizing the breath with the movement.

Spiritual – on swadhisthana chakra.

Sequence: This asana gives maximum benefits if preceded or followed by a forward bending asana. It may also be performed in conjunction with shalabhasana and dhanurasana for effective general health of the back and spine.

Contra-indications: People suffering from peptic ulcer, hernia, intestinal tuberculosis or hyperthyroidism should not practise this asana without the guidance of a competent teacher.

Benefits: This asana deepens breathing. It can help to remove backache and keep the spine supple and healthy. It tones the ovaries and uterus, and helps in gynaecological disorders. It stimulates appetite, alleviates constipation and is beneficial for all the abdominal organs, especially the liver and kidneys.

For cancer patients: People with metastases in the vertebral column should not practise this asana.

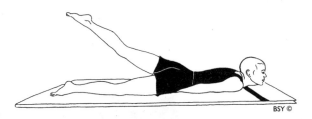

Ardha Shalabhasana (half locust pose)

Lie flat on the stomach with the hands under the thighs, palms downwards or hands clenched.

Keep both the legs straight throughout the practice.

Place the chin on the floor, slightly stretched forward, to give the best possible stretch to the neck muscles and nerves.

Using the back muscles, raise the left leg as high as possible, keeping the other leg straight, relaxed and in contact with the floor.

Retain the position for as long as is possible without strain. Do not tilt or twist the pelvis.

Lower the leg to the floor.

Repeat the same movement with the right leg.

This is one round.

Breathing: Inhale in the starting position.

Retain the breath inside while raising the leg and in the final position.

Exhale while lowering the leg to the starting position.

Duration: Up to 5 rounds when performed dynamically. Up to 3 rounds when performed statically.

Awareness: Physical – on the lower back, abdomen and heart, and on synchronizing the breath with the movement. Spiritual – on swadhisthana chakra.

Benefits: Ardha shalabhasana is an excellent asana for the back and pelvic organs. It can release tension in the pelvic area.

Practice note: The left leg should be raised first so that pressure is applied on the right side of the abdomen to massage the ascending colon of the large intestine, following the direction of intestinal peristalsis.

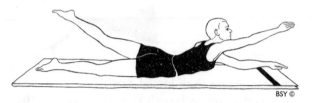

Variation: Lie on the stomach with the legs and feet together and the forehead touching the floor.

Stretch both arms above the head in advasana. Place the chin on the floor.

Keep the arms and legs straight throughout the practice. Simultaneously, raise the left leg, the head and right arm as high as possible.

The left leg should be stretched backwards and the right arm stretched forward as they are raised.

Retain the position for as long as possible without straining.

Lower the leg, head and arm to the starting position.

Relax in advasana, allowing the respiration to return to normal.

Repeat the same movement with the right leg and left arm.

This is one round. Practise up to 5 rounds.

Breathing: Inhale while raising the leg, arm and head.

Retain while holding the position.

Exhale while lowering the leg, arm and head to the starting position.

Awareness: Physical – on synchronizing the breath with the movement and on the diagonal stretch through the body from the tips of the toes of the raised leg to the fingertips of the opposite hand.

Spiritual – on swadhisthana chakra.

Benefits: This variation is beneficial for beginners with weak and stiff backs as it helps to tone the back muscles and stimulate the nerves, particularly in the lower back, while simultaneously giving a strong diagonal stretch to the body. It develops concentration through awareness of coordination of movement with breath.

For cancer patients: People with cancer of the pelvic organs or colon should not practise this asana.

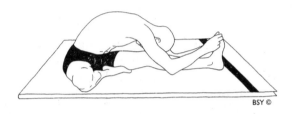

BSY ©

Janu Sirshasana (head to knee pose)

Sit with the legs outstretched and the feet together.

Bend the left leg, placing the heel of the foot against the perineum and the sole of the foot against the inside of the right thigh. Keep the left knee on the floor.

Place the hands on top of the right knee, keeping the spine straight and the back muscles relaxed.

This is the starting position.

Slowly bend forward, sliding the hands down the right leg, and grasp the right foot. If possible, hold the big toe with the index finger, middle finger and thumb of the left hand and the outside edge of the foot with the right hand.

Try to touch the knee with the forehead.

This is the final position.

Keep the back relaxed and do not strain.

Hold the position for as long as is comfortable.

Return to the starting position and rest the hands on the knees.

Change sides and repeat with the right leg bent and the left leg straight.

Practise up to 5 times with each leg.

Breathing: Inhale in the starting position.

Exhale while bending forward.

Retain the breath outside if holding the final position for a short time.

Breathe normally if holding the pose for a longer time.

Inhale while returning to the starting position.

Duration: Beginners may practise up to 5 rounds, staying in the final position for a short while. Adepts may practise only one round, but maintain the final position for up to 5 minutes.

Awareness: Physical – on the abdomen, relaxation of the back muscles, stretching of hamstring muscles at the back of the thigh, and on breathing.

Sequence: Before or after backward bending asanas.

Contra-indications: People with slipped disc or sciatica should not practise this asana without the guidance of an expert.

Benefits: This practice loosens up the legs in preparation for meditation asanas. It tones and massages the abdominal and pelvic organs, relaxes the back muscles and makes the back more supple. It gives the same benefits as paschimottanasana to a lesser degree.

Eka Pada Pranamasana (one-legged prayer pose)

Stand upright with the feet together and the arms at the sides. Focus the gaze on a fixed point in front of the body.

Bend the right leg, grasp the ankle and place the sole of the foot on the inside of the left thigh. The heel should be close to the perineum and the right knee should point out to the side.

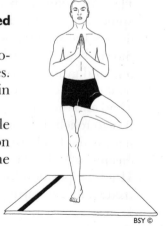

BSY ©

When the body is balanced, place the hands in prayer position in front of the chest for the final position.

Release the hands and then the foot.

Relax completely in the starting position, and change sides.

Breathing: Breathe normally throughout the practice.

Duration: Practise up to 3 rounds on each leg, holding the final position for up to 2 minutes.

Awareness: Physical – on a fixed point at eye level.

Spiritual – on ajna or anahata chakra.

Benefits: This asana develops nervous balance. It also strengthens the leg, ankle and foot muscles.

Variation: Assume the final position of eka pada pranamasana.

Keeping the gaze focused at eye level, inhale and raise the arms above the head, palms together. Hold the position with the breath inside and, on exhalation, lower the hands back in front of the chest. Repeat on the other side.

For cancer patients: Fragile people or those who cannot maintain balance should not practise this asana.

SHATKARMA

Jala Neti (nasal cleansing with water)

Preparation: A special *neti lota*, or neti pot, should be used. This pot may be made of plastic, pottery, brass or any other metal which does not contaminate the water. The nozzle on the end of the spout should fit comfortably into the nostril so that the water does not leak out. Even a teapot may be used if the tip of the spout is not too large or sharp.

The water should be pure, at body temperature and thoroughly mixed with salt in the proportion of one teaspoonful per half litre of water. The addition of salt ensures the osmotic pressure of the water is equal to that of the body fluids, thereby minimizing any irritation to the mucous membrane. A painful or burning sensation is an indication of too little or too much salt in the water.

Stage 1: Washing the nostrils

Fill the neti pot with the prepared salt water.

Stand squarely, with legs apart so that the body weight is evenly distributed between the feet. Lean forward and tilt the head to one side.

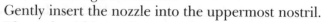

Breathe through the mouth.

Gently insert the nozzle into the uppermost nostril. There should be no force involved.

The nozzle should press firmly against the side of the nostril so that no water leakage occurs.

Tilt the neti pot in such a way that the water runs into the nostril and not down the face.

Keep the mouth open. Raising the elbow of the hand which holds the neti pot helps to adjust the body position so that the water flows out through the lower nostril.

When half the water has passed through the nostrils, remove the nozzle from the nostril, centre the head and let the water run out of the nose.

Remove any mucus from the nose by blowing gently.

Tilt the head to the opposite side and repeat the process, placing the nozzle of the lota in the upper nostril.

After completing this process, the nostrils must be thoroughly dried.

Stage 2: Drying the nostrils

1. Stand erect.

Close the right nostril with the right thumb and breathe in and out through the left nostril 10 times in quick succession, as in kapalbhati pranayama.

Repeat through the right nostril, with the left nostril closed. Perform once more through both nostrils.

2. Bend forward from the waist so that the trunk is horizontal. Repeat the same process as described above, but tilt the head to the right, closing the right nostril.

Repeat again, tilting the head to the left and closing the left nostril.

Finally, repeat again with the head centred, breathing through both nostrils.

Practice note: This step helps to drain trapped water from the sinus cavities.

3. Stand erect with the feet apart. Close the right nostril and exhale forcefully while bending forward rapidly from the waist. Inhale normally while returning to the upright position. Repeat 5 times.

Repeat with the right nostril open and then with both nostrils open. Do not blow the nose too hard as the remaining water may be pushed into the ears.

If necessary, perform shashankasana for several minutes to allow the drainage of any remaining water.

Duration: This practice should take about 5 minutes.

Neti may be practised daily, once or twice a week, or as required.

Awareness: Physical – on relaxing and positioning the body, on the flow of water through the nostrils, and on relaxed breathing through the mouth, especially for beginners.

Spiritual – on ajna chakra.

Sequence: Jala neti is ideally practised in the morning before asanas and pranayamas. However, if necessary, it may be performed at any time, except after meals.

Precautions: The water should only pass through the nostrils. If any water enters the throat or mouth it causes no harm, but indicates that the position of the head needs to be adjusted.

Make sure that the nose is properly dried after the practice, otherwise the nasal passages and sinuses may become irritated and manifest the symptoms of a cold.

Only practise neti when necessary. Prolonged practise is not advisable unless instructed by a competent teacher.

Contra-indications: People who suffer from chronic bleeding in the nose should not do jala neti without the advice of a competent teacher. Those who consistently have great difficulty passing water through the nose may have a structural blockage and should seek expert advice. People prone to or having ear infections should not do neti. During colds, flu or sinusitis, when the nose is totally blocked, neti should be avoided.

Benefits: Jala neti removes mucus and pollution from the nasal passages and sinuses, allowing air to flow without obstruction. It helps prevent and manage respiratory tract diseases. It helps to maintain good health of the ears, eyes and throat.

Jala neti relieves muscular tension of the face and helps the practitioner to maintain a fresh and youthful appearance. It has a calming and soothing influence on the brain. It alleviates anxiety, anger and depression, removes drowsiness and makes the head feel light and fresh.

Jala neti stimulates the various nerve endings in the nose, improving the sense of smell and the overall health of the individual. A balance is brought about between the right and left nostrils and the corresponding left and right brain hemispheres, inducing a state of harmony and balance throughout the body and mind. Most importantly, however, jala neti helps to awaken ajna chakra.

For cancer patients: People with cancer in the head, face and neck regions should not practise jala neti. People with impaired swallowing should also not practise jala neti.

Practice note: Jala neti may be practised either in a squatting position or standing. The latter is most suitable for doing neti over a sink while the former may be performed outside. After some practice, a full neti pot may be used for each nostril.

Variations: Practitioners may suck water up the nostrils directly from a glass or bowl. This is the original form of the practice called *vyutkrama kapalbhati*, or *usha paan*, which literally means 'water of the dawn'.

Kunjal Kriya (the practice of vomiting water)

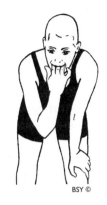

Wash the hands and make sure the nails are carefully trimmed. Prepare 2 litres of warm salted water as described in the practice of jala neti.

Stand near a sink or toilet, or if the weather is warm, in a suitable place outside in the garden or near an open drain.

Drink at least 6 glasses of the prepared lukewarm salted water, one after the other, as quickly as possible, until the stomach cannot hold any more. It is most important to drink fast and not just sip the water.

When the stomach is full, the urge to vomit will occur automatically.

Lean forward, keeping the trunk as horizontal as possible.

Open the mouth and place the middle and index fingers of the right hand as far back on the tongue as possible.

Gently rub and press the back of the tongue.

This should induce the water to gush out from the stomach. If there is no expulsion of water, it means the tips of the fingers are not far enough down the throat or that the tongue is not being pressed.

The more the practitioner relaxes into the practice, the easier it will be.

During the expulsion of water the fingers may be removed from the mouth, although this is not necessary.

When the flow of water ceases, again place the fingers in the mouth and repeat the process.

Continue in this way until the stomach is empty.

Practice note: Plain water may be used on the advice of a yoga teacher. Salt water, however, dissolves mucus and also inhibits the secretion of acid in the stomach, making it generally preferable, and a must for those suffering from excess mucus and hyperacidity.

Some people are unable to bring up the water at first. The water in the stomach will then simply pass through the

211

system in the normal way. The biggest obstacle is the mental block people have towards the idea of vomiting.

The expelled water may be discoloured initially due to fermented food particles, bile or mucus from the stomach. When the stomach is completely clean the water will become clear.

Time of practice: Kunjal kriya is done early in the morning before breakfast. However, if it is very cold it is better to wait until the day has warmed up a little. It is essential that no food is taken before the practice.

Frequency: Once a week is sufficient for most people.

Precaution: When the vomiting reflex ceases to bring up any water, stop the practice as this is a sure sign that the stomach is empty. The practice removes some of the stomach lining, leaving it temporarily vulnerable. For this reason it is advisable not to eat until half an hour after completion of the practice.

Sequence: It should be followed by jala neti.

Contra-indications: It should not be practised by people suffering from hernia, high blood pressure, raised intracranial pressure, heart disease, stroke, acute peptic ulcer or diabetics with eye problems.

Benefits: Indigestion, acidity and gas can be overcome. Excess mucus is removed from the body, helping to remedy cough and cold, bronchitis, asthma and other respiratory ailments. Bad breath is eradicated.

It also helps to release pent-up emotions and emotional blocks or feelings of heaviness in the heart caused by inner and external conflict and pressures.

For cancer patients: People with cancer of the head, face, neck and chest regions and of the oesophagus and stomach should not practise kunjal kriya. Debilitated and frail people should also refrain from it. People with primary or metastatic cancer in the brain should not attempt it. Those with prolonged bleeding or clotting time, or blood cancer should not do kunjal kriya. People with advanced cancer of an abdominal organ, recent abdominal surgery or chemotherapy or radiotherapy should refrain from it.

Laghoo Shankhaprakshalana (short intestinal wash)

Prepare two litres of warm salted water as described in the practice of jala neti.

Quickly drink 2 glasses of the prepared water.

Perform the following 5 asanas dynamically 8 times each:

a) Tadasana
b) Tiryaka tadasana
c) Kati chakrasana (variation)
d) Tiryaka bhujangasana
e) Udarakarshanasana.

Drink 2 more glasses of water and repeat the asanas 8 times each.

Repeat the process for a third and last time.

Go to the toilet, but do not strain, whether there is a bowel movement or not.

If there is no motion immediately, it will come later on.

Additional practices: Kunjal kriya and jala neti may be performed immediately after completing the practice.

Time of practice: Laghoo should be practised in the morning when the stomach is completely empty, before any food or drink is taken.

Duration: Allow an hour for this practice.

Frequency: Once a week is sufficient for general purposes. In cases of constipation, however, it may be practised daily until the condition improves.

Rest: On completion of the practice, rest for half an hour before taking any food or drink.

Restrictions: There are no special food restrictions and no special food has to be taken following this practice, although a light vegetarian diet is preferable for that day.

Precautions: Do not try to force a bowel movement; it should be completely natural.

Contra-indications: People with high blood pressure, heart disease, impaired kidney function and all those whose salt intake is restricted should not practise it. People with colitis or ulcers in the colon should avoid this practice in the acute phase. It is a strenuous practice and should not be attempted by elderly, debilitated or frail people in low energy states. It should not be practised for three months after major surgery, and for six months if the surgery involved the oesophagus, stomach, intestines, colon or rectum.

Benefits: Laghoo alleviates digestive disorders such as indigestion, gas, acidity and constipation, and tones the liver and other digestive glands. It is helpful in diabetes, in obesity, and for high cholesterol and triglycerides in the blood. This practice flushes and stimulates the kidneys. It purifies the blood by encouraging the excretion of waste products and toxins, which assists in skin conditions. It assists in the management of asthma by reducing excess mucus. Laghoo strengthens the immune system, relives symptoms of arthritis, and reduces mental and emotional stress. At the pranic level it recharges the whole pranamaya kosha by removing blockages from the nadis and stimulates the chakras.

For cancer patients: Cancer patients who have successfully completed chemotherapy and radiotherapy, for whom three months has passed after surgery (six months in the case of surgery on the digestive system) and whose general health is stable can practise it once a fortnight to strengthen the immune system and to encourage the excretion of the residue of drugs from the body.

People with cancer of the digestive tract should not do this practice before surgical removal of the growth. It should not be practised during or soon after chemotherapy or radiotherapy as the internal tissues are very fragile and may be damaged. It is advisable to wait for 4-6 weeks after the last cycle of treatment.

Practice note: Greater benefits may be derived by combining this practice with light food. Medication may be safely continued.

Alternative mini-scale technique: TTK solution

One litre of warm salted water should be prepared, or pure unsalted water at room temperature can be used if the weather is not too cold.

The first three asanas of the shankhaprakshalana series are used:

a) Tadasana

b) Tiryaka tadasana

c) Kati chakrasana (variation)

Quickly drink one glass of the prepared water.

Practise tadasana 10 times and drink a second glass of water.

Practise tiryaka tadasana 10 times and drink a third glass of water.

Practise kati chakrasana 10 times and drink a fourth glass of water.

Go to the toilet, but do not strain, whether there is a bowel movement or not. If there is no motion immediately, it will come later on.

Time of practice: The TTK solution should be practised in the morning when the stomach is completely empty, before any food or drink is taken and before other asanas.

Frequency: Once a week is sufficient for general purposes. In cases of constipation, however, it can be practised daily until the condition improves.

Restrictions: There are no special food restrictions and no special food has to be taken following this practice.

Precautions: Do not try to force a bowel movement; it should be completely natural.

Benefits: This practice helps to prevent constipation and related digestive problems. It makes the body feel light and ensures a healthy intake of water first thing in the morning.

DHARANA

Sadbhavana meditation (goodwill meditation)

This meditation can be practised at the end of the spiritual practice session, at the end of the meditation practice, at the end of the day, whenever emotionally disturbed or whenever the urge is felt.

Technique

Sit comfortably in a meditative asana of your choice with the spine straight, but without any tension. Place your hands be on the knees or in the lap in a mudra of your choice. Close your eyes gently. Allow your consciousness to move from one part of your body to another briskly, in a sequence, starting from the toes and going all the way up to the head, making any adjustments necessary for total comfort and relaxation. *Pause.*

Your body is now comfortable, firm and motionless. Take your awareness to your natural breath. Closely watch each ingoing and outgoing breath. *Pause.* Your breath is slowly becoming slower and more subtle. *Pause.*

Let your awareness flow into your chest, riding on the in-breath. Allow your awareness to settle on the innermost point that your breath is touching. *Pause.* Now feel peaceful and calm. Allow the sensation of peace to flood the whole of the heart space. See it in the form of a calm, deep ocean. *Pause.* Feel at ease, at harmony, within. *Pause.* Feel joy and happiness. *Pause.* Experience these feelings in the form of the gentle waves of the ocean and see yourself swimming in this ocean. *Pause.*

Chant the Shanti mantras mentally, slowly, with understanding. *Asato maa sadgamaya. Pause. Tamaso maa jyotirgamaya. Pause. Mrityor maamritam gamaya. Pause.* Visualize many other people swimming in the ocean of your heart space, hridayakasha. They are people whom you know and can identify, or whom you do not know; people whom you like or dislike, young and old, men and

216

women. *Pause.* Send them your heartfelt good wishes by continuing the mantras as before. *Sarveshaam svastirbhavatu. Pause. Sarveshaam shantirbhavatu. Pause. Sarveshaam poornam bhavatu. Pause. Sarveshaam mangalam bhavatu. Pause. Lokaah samastaah sukhino bhavantu. Pause.* Pray for the wellbeing of the whole universe, all living beings and non-living things. *Om tryambakam yajaamahe, sugandhim pushti-vardhanam, urvaarukamiva bandhanaat, mrityormuksheeya mamritaat. Om shaantih shaantih shaantih. Pause.* Visualize your ishta deva in hridayakasha. *Pause.* Bowing to him, continue the chant. *Tvameva maataa cha pitaa tvameva, tvameva bandhushcha sakhaa tvameva, tvameva vidyaa dravinam tvameva, tvameva sarvam mama deva deva. Tvameva sarvam mama deva deva, tvameva sarvam mama deva deva. Hari Om.*

Sit quietly for some time. *Pause.* Let the image of your ishta deva dissolve. *Pause.* Become aware of your body, the whole body in the meditative posture. Become aware of your natural breath. *Pause.* Gradually externalize your mind by observing the state of mind, the various sensations generated within and on the surface of your body. *Pause.* Allow the awareness to expand by observing the external atmosphere, its sounds, smell, touch and light sensations. *Pause.* When you are ready, start moving the body, rub your palms together and place the warm palms over the closed eyes. Gently open your eyes.

Hari Om Tat Sat

8

Management of Bothering Conditions

PHYSICAL

When cancer establishes itself in the body, its effects eventually begin to manifest. Some of the effects are due to a *disruption in the normal functioning of the organ*. The cancer cells compete for space and nutrients with normal tissue, causing some impairment of functioning, depending on the stage of its growth. In advanced stages it can completely take over, leading to total failure of the organ. Indigestion, bloating, constipation, irregular bowel habit, persistent cough, muscular weakness and visual disturbances are some of the commonly found symptoms due to impaired organ function. Both conventional medical treatment and yoga practices are well geared to manage these effects. Home remedies and alternative therapies also have a lot to offer in this area.

As the cancer area increases in size, it also exerts *pressure on neighbouring tissues*, causing local symptoms. This results in different symptoms, depending on the tissue where pressure is applied. If pressure is being placed on the skin, a lump may develop; if it is being placed on the liver or its surroundings, then jaundice can occur. Pressure on the vocal cords can cause hoarseness of the voice. These symptoms can only be relieved by shrinking the cancer. Hence, the conventional medical treatments are most effective in dealing with them.

Pain is a relatively common feature of cancer. In some cancers it is delayed until very advanced stages, while in others it is one of the earliest symptoms. Pain can be caused by pressure on the nerves, swelling or inflammation in affected organs, lack of adequate blood supply, release of irritant toxins, or actual degeneration of the cancer or normal cells. It could also be due to surgery, radiotherapy or other cancer treatments. Pain is generally the most distressing symptom, and pain relief is a very important aspect of cancer management. Modern medicine has many tools of varying magnitude in its arsenal to combat this symptom. Yoga and alternative or complementary therapies also offer substantial relief, sometimes using much simpler means.

Cancer cells multiply at an enormous speed. They are voracious consumers of nutrients and they successfully compete with normal cells. Comparative starvation of the healthy cells of the body causes symptoms of fatigue, generalized weakness and unexplained loss of weight. The toxins (products of metabolism) released by the cancerous cells may be responsible for malaise (lack of wellbeing), loss of appetite, nausea, low-grade fever and poor digestion. Yoga, by working on the *prana*, the energy system of the body, can relieve many of these symptoms considerably.

If surgical treatment, chemotherapy or radiotherapy has been given then there will likely be *side effects*, adding to the existing physical suffering. The most common of these symptoms are pain, extreme weakness, poor appetite, diarrhoea, persistent nausea, vomiting, hair loss, loss of a body part or organ, and impairment of the immune system (inability to fight against infection). Fortunately, most of these symptoms are transient and wear off as the body heals or the therapeutic agent is excreted from the body. Both yoga and medical science offer valuable tools to help manage this difficult time.

Common bothering physical conditions are:
• Pain, including burning pain
• Loss of appetite
• Nausea and vomiting

- Indigestion, flatulence and heartburn
- Constipation and diarrhoea
- Weakness and fatigue
- Sleep disturbances
- Shortness of breath
- Restricted movement
- Swelling
- Scarring or amputation, hair loss.

DEALING WITH PHYSICAL CONDITIONS

1. Pain

Pain has many causes. It is a warning sign coming from the body telling us that something is wrong, please attend to it. Pain should not be neglected. Very often the cause can be addressed. One should try to do so by all available means. If the cause is beyond our reach or is transitory, medical experts usually suggest pain relieving drugs.

When a new pain starts, ask yourself a few questions. When did it start? What were you doing then? What type of pain is it – throbbing, dull aching, shooting, burning? Where is it? Spreading somewhere or localized? What makes it worse? What eases it? Have you experienced similar pain before? Report to your doctor and follow his advice. After consultation, if you are convinced that it is only transitory, or there is no curative remedy and the doctor can only advise pain relieving drugs, you may like to try yoga or other simple methods. They can be used along with the doctor's medication to optimize the medication's effectiveness and/or enable less dependence on medication.

Please remember that there is *no need to endure pain*. It must be duly attended to.

Yoga: Regular practice of a balanced yoga program will reduce pain by helping to remove the pain-producing and harmful chemicals, and releasing chemicals that are responsible for our sense of wellbeing. For immediate relief of pain, however, try one of the following.

220

- Practise staying still and relaxing the body with full awareness. Particularly relax the painful area. Then take your awareness to the breath. Observe it intently. Allow it to become slow, deep and rhythmic. Count the breaths. Practise for a few minutes or for as long as you are comfortable. The practice will become more effective as you gain experience.
- In acute pain, rest the affected area. If you need to move that part, then do so gently and cautiously. Once the acute phase is over, then start mobilizing the area gradually. This will release the stiffness and improve the circulation of prana and blood, giving pain relief. Asanas from the pawanmuktasana part I series and spinal stretching asanas such as tadasana, tiryaka tadasana, kati chakrasana and marjari-asana are very effective.
- Find a comfortable posture that minimizes pain by experimenting with relaxing asanas combined with breath awareness, e.g. matsya kridasana, advasana or makarasana with the feet comfortably apart, shashankasana, shavasana.
- Practise yoga nidra. Deep muscular relaxation will relieve pain due to reactionary muscle spasm. Mental relaxation will allow the mind to be moved from its attachment to a painful area. Yoga nidra will train the person to go beyond the sensation of pain. The pain remains, but the person does not feel so affected by it, and learns to accept, adjust and live with it. This state of relaxation actually produces chemicals in the body that promote healing, thus removing the cause of pain.
- Practise ajapa japa. Find a comfortable sitting, semi-reclined or lying posture. Introvert your awareness by first observing the parts of your body in a sequence and then observing the normal breath. Then shift your awareness to the psychic breath between the navel and the throat. Continue for as long as you can comfortably. You may choose to use the mantra *Soham* or your personal mantra with psychic breathing. Alternatively you can use any other psychic passage.

- Focus your mind on mantra japa or mantra chanting, or practise a dharana practice of your choice.

Other remedies: Massage, or using an ice pack or a heat pack are helpful in different situations. Do not massage the area directly over the tumour or metastasis. Refrain from massage for a few weeks after surgery and consult your doctor before starting it. Avoid applying heat on irradiated areas and surgical wounds. Do not use an ice pack just before exercise. Magnet therapy and pranic healing may offer help.

2. Loss of appetite and nausea

The harmful products of metabolism released by cancerous cells may be responsible for malaise or lack of wellbeing, loss of appetite and nausea. Surgery, chemotherapy, radiotherapy or other drugs can also produce loss of appetite and nausea. A changed taste in the mouth can lead to a dislike of food. Fearful, depressed or anxious states of mind can also produce aversion to food.

Yoga: A basic and balanced yoga program will help relieve these symptoms. The following practices will provide further assistance. Drink two or three glasses of plain water early in the morning on an empty stomach and perform tadasana, tiryaka tadasana, kati chakrasana and supta pawanmuktasana five times each. Asanas from the pawanmuktasana part 2 series are also very helpful. If the cancer is affecting any abdominal organs, then avoid asanas that compress the abdomen.

Kunjal kriya and laghoo shankhaprakshalana are also very good, provided the practitioner has enough stamina to do them. If the cancer is affecting the digestive system or the brain, then refrain from these practices. In the case of head, neck and lung cancer avoid kunjal kriya. People with ulcers in the digestive system, impaired kidney function, hypertension, heart disease and glaucoma should not do these practices. Wait for at least six months if you have undergone any surgery.

General measures: Try a liquid diet instead of a solid one, or eat easily digestible food instead of rich food, and have small portions of food in place of large amounts. Use spices and condiments like cumin, coriander, ginger, anise, dandelion, black pepper and mint that aid digestion. Fresh lemon juice half an hour before a meal is a good idea. The spices and the lemon stimulate the secretion of digestive juices in the body.

3. Digestive problems (indigestion, gas, heartburn, diarrhoea)

Improper diet, wrong eating habits, inadequate functioning of the digestive system because of cancer, inadequate physical movement, an unhappy mind, chemotherapy and radio-therapy, and the use of certain other medications can lead to these symptoms. Such symptoms may be pre-existing irrespective of the cancer.

Yoga: All the tips that are useful for loss of appetite and nausea also apply to these symptoms.

Other remedies: Papaya fruit, including the seeds, is beneficial. Half a teaspoon of commercially prepared aloe vera juice taken before a meal can be beneficial. Do not combine it with any laxative or diuretic. Aloe vera gel obtained by cutting a fresh leaf is different to the juice, and only for external application.

General measures: Avoid too little or too much food. Avoid lying down just after eating. Keep the evening meal light and avoid a late dinner. Take proteins and fats in smaller amounts and in forms that are easily digestible. Some fruit and vegetable juices can produce gas or acidity. In such cases, it is advised to cook the vegetables and either eat the fruits whole or totally avoid them. One school of thought believes that cold milk is not useful in combating acidity in the long term. It gives immediate relief, but may increase acid secretion in the stomach after a time lapse as a rebound action. So discuss it with your doctor.

4. Constipation

The cause can be insufficient or incorrect diet, inadequate fluid intake, medication-induced, a pre-existing condition, cancer either directly involving the digestive system or pressing on it from outside, and inadequate physical movement and activity. Depression, worries and fear can contribute to constipation.

Yoga: Drink one to one and a half litres of plain water early in the morning on an empty stomach and perform tadasana, tiryaka tadasana, kati chakrasana and supta pawanmuktasana five times each. Asanas from the pawan-muktasana part 2 series are also very helpful. If the cancer is affecting any of the abdominal organs, then avoid asanas that compress the abdomen.

Laghoo shankhaprakshalana is also very beneficial, provided the practitioner has enough stamina to do it. If the cancer is affecting the digestive system or the brain, then refrain from this practice. People with ulcers in the digestive system, impaired kidney function, hypertension, heart disease and glaucoma should not practise it.

General measures: Correct the diet and increase physical activity as much as possible. Ensure adequate fibre content in the food you are eating. The chief sources of fibre are fresh fruits with skin, whole grains, oatmeal, bran, and vegetables. Drink enough water, about two and a half to three litres per day. If possible, replace the constipation-causing drug with a more suitable one.

Avoid coffee, tea, other caffeinated drinks and alcohol as they are diuretics and will increase dehydration. Avoid binding foods such as bananas, rice, peeled apples and dry toast. Sugary foods also tend to cause constipation.

5. Weakness and fatigue

Cancer cells consume nutrients voraciously and they successfully compete with normal cells. Comparative starvation of the body's healthy cells causes fatigue, generalized weakness and unexplained loss of weight. The toxic products of metabolism released by the cancerous cells may also be responsible for weakness and fatigue. Inability to eat or digest food properly can also contribute to weakness and fatigue. Depression and other negative states of mind may be additional factors.

Yoga: Regular yoga practice can be a great help in managing this problem. Yoga works on the energy system or prana. It mobilizes stagnant energy and also helps to generate extra prana. It lifts depression, settles anxiety and alleviates fear, thus elevating the energy level. Asanas from the pawanmuktasana part 1 series are very helpful, along with tadasana, tiryaka tadasana and kati chakrasana.

Deep, slow breathing or yogic breathing, nadi shodhana pranayama and, if possible, bhastrika pranayama at a slow speed may be practised. Yoga nidra is a highly rejuvenating practice for cancer patients. Meditation practices such as ajapa japa and trataka generate fresh energy, helping to relieve fatigue and generalized weakness.

General measures: Avoid either excessive or inadequate resting – try to find a balance between resting too much and too little. Give your body time to recover from treatment. More than usual rest is needed after surgery/chemotherapy/radiotherapy for the body to recover properly. Stay mobile as much as possible. At the same time do not overstrain. Pay attention to your diet. Make sure it is not deficient. Regulate your lifestyle.

6. Sleep disturbances

The toxic products of the metabolic processes of cancerous cells and the destruction of cancer cells by chemotherapy drugs and radioactive agents may cause an inability to sleep. Fear, tension, depression and other mental states may prevent relaxation and subsequent drifting into sleep. Pain and other uncomfortable symptoms can also prevent sleep or cause waking up in the middle of sleep. Improper eating times, especially a heavy dinner taken late, and gas or indigestion may also impair sleep.

Yoga: Practise yoga regularly. Regular practice of asana, pranayama and especially meditative practices is miraculous in normalizing sleep patterns. Practising yoga nidra regularly alleviates anxiety and fear, releases accumulated stress and makes the mind calm and peaceful. This improves the sleep pattern. Yoga nidra also provides deep relaxation, thus partially compensating for inadequate physical and mental rest due to insomnia. Practise mantra japa and chanting regularly. Both the physical and mental energies are balanced by yoga practices, inducing a relaxed state.

When you retire at night, practise breath awareness, bhramari pranayama, trataka on a jyoti or candle flame, and go to bed repeating your personal mantra or keeping your awareness on the breath. Alternatively, do yoga nidra when you go to bed.

Other remedies: Take sleep-inducing medication or soothing substances if absolutely necessary. They may be helpful for a limited time. Herbal teas such as chamomile, passionflower, valerian or hops can be soothing before bedtime. Before taking any remedy, including herbal products, be sure you know its potential side effects.

General measures: Maintain regular hours of sleeping irrespective of the quality and quantity of sleep. Make sure you are not too cold or too hot, that your clothing is comfortably loose and of natural fibre, the bed is comfortable, your pillow is comfortable and the right size and the room is cool, quiet and dark. Have a warm bath before sleeping. Take adequate pain-relieving measures before bedtime. Use your bed only for sleeping. Do not work, watch TV, read or eat in bed. The aroma of lavender oil in the bedroom can help to induce sleep.

Regulate eating times and the content of the diet to suit your body's constitution. Eat early, preferably at sunset or at least three hours prior to bedtime. Have a very light dinner. Restrict protein and fat content to as much as you can digest. Avoid large meals even if they are easily digestible.

If frequent urination is disturbing sleep, then regulate the fluid intake after sunset and change the time of medication or other substances (such as alcohol) that encourage urine production. Discuss this symptom with your doctor if it persists.

Change the time of medication and/or restrict the intake of other substances (such as coffee) that stimulate the nervous system. Have as much physical activity as possible during the day, but avoid excessive exertion during the evening, as this will stimulate wakefulness. If necessary, minimize daytime sleeping. Engage in enjoyable activities to change any negative mindset. Spend time in the fresh air, and in the company of happy people or children.

7. Shortness of breath

Pressure of a tumour on respiratory organs, cancer directly involving the respiratory system, fluid retention from any cause, anaemia, pre-existing respiratory or cardiac conditions, and large amounts of radiotherapy to the chest are some of the common causes of shortness of breath. The presence of pain, recent surgery or gas in the digestive system can also hamper breathing. Fear, anxiety or an emotionally-charged state of mind can aggravate the problem.

Yoga: Practise breath awareness. Breathe in deeply and slowly. Practise abdominal breathing. Asanas such as hasta utthanasana which expand the chest are beneficial. Practise nadi shodhana pranayama in the ratio of 1:1 or 1:2, gradually increasing the count; for example, 5:5 to 6:6 to 7:7, or 4:8 to 5:10 to 6:12. Practise ujjayi pranayama. Awareness of the ujjayi breath moving in a psychic passage, as in ajapa japa, is even more beneficial. The mantra *Soham* or your personal mantra can be used simultaneously. Prana mudra and mudra breathing are also useful. For details refer to *Yoga Darshan*, published by Yoga Publications Trust.

General measures: If it is a new symptom or an old one recurring after a long time, then report it to your doctor. Attend to treatable causes if any, such as pain, an overloaded abdomen, or digestive gas. Any measure that relieves stress is helpful.

8. Restricted movements

This can be due to temporary injury to muscles or joints as a result of surgical handling of the tissues. Depending on the condition, the area should generally be rested for around 48 hours and then gradually mobilized. An expert (such as a physiotherapist) can be consulted if there is doubt. Application of heat or cold is a simple but effective remedy.

Yoga: Gradually start mobilizing the area, using appropriate asanas. The pawanmuktasana part 1 series, tadasana, tiryaka tadasana, kati chakrasana, marjari-asana and supta udarakarshanasana are some of the most useful ones. Breath awareness, slow deep breathing and soothing pranayamas like bhramari and nadi shodhana are helpful as they relax the area of tension. Yoga nidra with a healing visualization of the area concerned can help to bring about a fast and complete recovery. Mentally visualizing movement of the area in fine detail is equally beneficial.

9. Swelling

This can occur as a result of an inflammatory reaction to surgical handling of the tissue. The area should be rested for 48 hours. Elevation above heart level and the application of heat or cold are simple but effective remedies.

Yoga: Gradually start mobilizing the area using appropriate asanas. The pawanmuktasana part 1 series, tadasana, tiryaka tadasana, kati chakrasana, marjari-asana and supta udarakarshanasana are some of the useful ones.

10. Scarring or amputation, hair loss

These can be quite traumatic, having a strong effect on one's self-image and confidence. Often the disfigurement is long term or permanent. External props or restorative surgery may be possible at a later date. Sometimes, however, there is no easy solution and it is only by developing the attitude of acceptance that peace can be felt. Very often, in order to gain something, something else has to be given up or let go of. At times we must choose a lesser evil in order to escape a greater evil. The mind tends to be good at accepting rational arguments, and so developing a clear understanding of the situation can be a great help in learning to accept change after an initial shock and attendant feelings of denial. This attitude also helps when we are faced with important decisions on future actions. The niyamas *santosha*, contentment, and *ishwara pranidhana*, faith in a higher reality, help us develop an attitude of acceptance and even gratitude. Such attitudes lift us out of self-pity and into positive states of mind and emotion.

11. Burning skin

Avoid heat, exposure to the sun, rubbing the area with any rough surface, soap or any chemical. Wear very loose and soft clothing. Aloe vera gel can bring relief. Sandalwood and turmeric paste can also be effective.

MENTAL

A diagnosis of cancer produces an emotional shock which causes disturbances in our mental functioning. If the cancer involves the brain, either primarily or as a result of its spread, then it can produce a direct and physiologically based imbalance in mental functions.

The mental function of *cognition* (understanding what is perceived) can become distorted for various reasons. Fear is a major one. Other common factors that may contribute to distortion in perception when a person is diagnosed with cancer include an incomplete understanding of the disease and of the life situation as a whole, pre-existing wrong beliefs, and a tendency to imagine and speculate (over- or under-assessment) about a situation, rather than depending on solid facts.

Some people lose *self-confidence and willpower*, perhaps only initially, when they learn about the presence of any major illness within. Once they adjust, they may recover from this emotional shock and show increased self-confidence and willpower, kindled by their survival instinct. However, some fail to recover their mental strength. They succumb to the fear of death and enter into the deep valley of self-pity and passive acceptance. This lack of self-confidence and willpower slowly percolates into every activity of daily life.

Some people lose interest in life and become *dull and introverted*. Their faculty of perception slows down, diminishing the ability to understand and integrate. Clarity in understanding can also deteriorate to some extent. Some people show *restlessness* due to am underlying metabolic imbalance or anxiety.

Diminished self-confidence, low or distorted perception and lack of clarity in understanding lead to *indecisiveness*. In these mental states an individual tends to postpone decision-making.

Yoga not only provides relief from the physical symptoms, but also relaxes the mind completely. With yoga practice, the mind becomes calm and receptive. The emotions also settle to some extent. With training in one-pointed awareness through yoga, clarity of mind is restored. The mind starts thinking rationally and making decisions confidently. People come out of their shell of hopelessness and depression and again take charge of their lives.

DEALING WITH MENTAL CONDITIONS

1. Poor concentration and difficulty in understanding

This limitation leads to difficulty in understanding the situation. It hampers the process of learning and acquiring new skills. It creates confusion in the mind. The mind is unable to make decisions promptly and correctly. Lack of mental clarity complicates all other issues of practical importance. Many unnecessary thoughts preoccupy the insecure and fearful mind. Such a mind jumps from one thought to another under the effect of rajas guna. At other times, under the effect of tamas guna, it withdraws into a shell and becomes totally unresponsive. In both of these states, the mind cannot be applied effectively to anything. It cannot concentrate on anything and therefore cannot grasp or understand. This compounds the feeling of insecurity.

Yoga: Through its ability to relax the mind, yoga awakens creativity, which is the ability to find a solution to an obstacle. Awareness of the breath, bhramari pranayama, nadi shodhana pranayama and yoga nidra are primary practices for inducing relaxation. Yoga re-establishes the power of focused awareness through concentration technique such as trataka, ajapa japa and mantra japa.

Yoga can help resolve the fear of death, suffering or uncertainty with the help of meditative practices according to the choice and preference of the individual. In the practice of antar mouna, the practitioner is guided to observe various thoughts and feelings as a *drashta*, or witness. In the hands of an adept or under the guidance of a skilled teacher, antar mouna is a very powerful practice to go to the root cause of fear and then to deal with that fear. Bhakti yoga can awaken our innate inner strength, which helps us face all fears. Self-analytical practices like SWAN sadhana can also be utilized for this purpose.

2. Low self-esteem

Feelings of guilt, fear and insecurity lead to low self-esteem. Physical limitations may add to poor self-confidence.

Yoga: The wonderful practice of yoga nidra provides the opportunity to work out these emotions. The power of these negative emotions can also be reduced by cultivating the opposite positive emotions of love or nurturing, or by the protection generated during *sadbhavana*, goodwill meditation, or by bhakti yoga. These negative emotions can also be dealt with in contemplative, self-analytical jnana yoga practices, using logic and intuition.

General measures: Having the correct information and knowledge about the disease dispels many misconceptions and helps people to clear these negative feelings and regain control over the situation. The loving support of a spouse, family member or close friend can play a vital role in healing the serious emotional jolt that a diagnosis of cancer brings. Seeking the appropriate support to deal with physical and emotional limitations as and when needed is an important part of the overall management of cancer and its more subtle effects.

3. Weak willpower

Lack of self-confidence weakens the willpower. When we learn to connect with the inner self with the help of dharana practices, our confidence, and with it our willpower, returns.

Yoga: Breath awareness is the first step towards re-establishing our connection with the inner self. Once we have laid a foundation with breath awareness, the dharana (concentration) practices of ajapa japa and trataka are the leading tools for this purpose. Yoga nidra is another useful tool for regaining willpower.

Bhakti yoga practices help to balance disturbed emotions. Particularly powerful bhakti practices are kirtan and mantra chanting (singing the glories of the Lord); mantra japa and anushthana (repeating His name); *shravana* (listening to His stories); *archana* (worshipping Him); and *satsang* (being in the company of saints and following their teachings). As the clouded mind becomes clear, access to the inner self becomes easier. In bhakti yoga it is essential to have faith in the Lord and to feel a relationship or bond with Him. *Bhava*, feeling, is the vehicle on which the *bhakta* or devotee, the practitioner, rides to meet the Lord.

EMOTIONAL

A diagnosis of cancer tips our emotional balance. The ongoing physical discomforts and suffering aggravate the imbalance.

The root cause behind the emotional upheavals that a person with cancer undergoes is the feeling of insecurity, *abhinivesha*. The person is not sure about their lifespan, the amount of suffering that is ahead, their own capacity to cope with it, the ability to cope with the additional financial burden and the future of family members who may be left behind. Through yoga, a person can regain their emotional balance.

232

Yoga can be the best counsellor and friend. Yoga helps one establish a link with the innermost core of one's being. This provides an unshakeable support to rely upon.

When the final diagnosis comes, the person feels as if they have been given a life sentence. The unknown and half known truths about the cancer itself, and also about death and life after death, generate a great amount of *fear and anxiety*. A correct and in-depth understanding of the disease and its process can solve many of the fears that arise due to misconceptions. Every cancer has its own course and the future is not always gloomy. In fact, with courage and a clear understanding, the future can be made much brighter. Similarly, spiritual guidance and practice can resolve many fears about suffering, the dying process, death and life after death. Yogic practices help clear the clouds of doubts, restore self-confidence and allow the bright sun of clarity in understanding the situation and deciding on coping strategies to shine in one's intellect. Yoga also allows the heart to open to an acceptance of that which is beyond one's capacity to know or to change.

Those whose minds are conditioned to the idea that 'good deeds lead to rewards and bad deeds lead to punishment' often develop a strong sense of *guilt*. Yogic spiritual practices help cleanse the conscious, subconscious and unconscious levels of the mind of this sense of guilt which often weighs heavily on one's heart, preventing inner peace. When unresolved, this sense of guilt can result in feelings of frustration and anger against oneself, family members or care-givers, society at large, or the higher self or God.

Insecurity, fear and guilt, along with the various physical discomforts of illness, can lead to loss of hope, despair and *depression*. The ability to connect with one'sbeloved God or the inner self through yogic practices provides strength and a feeling of peace and inner joy which lifts us out of our gloomy state of mind. It also helps re-establish lost confidence and faith in the higher self.

Difficulties and limitations experienced in performing daily routine jobs can be another trigger for difficult emotions. Waiting for test results, sitting outside the treatment room, undergoing treatment procedures, or being in a crowd can also trigger stress or difficult emotions.

Common emotional imbalances revolve around the emotional states of anxiety, depression, fear, guilt, self-pity, frustration and grief.

Fig. 8.1: Emotional and Mental Disturbances in Cancer

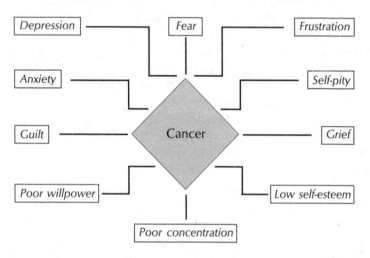

Dealing with Emotional Conditions

Yoga: A yogic lifestyle lived with awareness is the most simple and most basic step to stabilize our negative emotions. When the principle of regularity is staunchly followed, it does not allow any opportunity for long hours of mental brooding or day-dreaming. It forces us to go on with our responsibilities.

Watch and dissect the events that trigger your emotions. Very often the event under scrutiny is not the real cause. Find the source of the disturbance and address it directly. If necessary, express yourself adequately.

Regular practice of cleansing kriyas, asana and pranayama will mobilize the stagnant prana or energy and ensure its free flow throughout the body. Swami Niranjanananda describes emotion as energy in motion. Sudden, uncontrolled surges of pranic movement arising from anahata chakra in the heart area, and going to ajna chakra in the head area, where they hijack our wisdom, is emotion. Sometimes this uncontrolled movement originates very deep in the lower abdomen or pelvis, the area of swadhisthana or mooladhara chakra, then surges upward, shaking anahata and overpowering the intellect. When the nadis, the passages for the movement of prana, are obstructed, the prana bottles up and at a certain point, usually due to some trigger, it bursts out wildly in the form of emotion, whether positive or negative. Hatha yoga cleansing kriyas, asanas and pranayamas ensure unobstructed nadis and a free, smooth and controlled flow of physical energy (*prana shakti*), as well as mental energy (*chitta shakti*). This means a smooth, balanced flow of both physical and mental energy, leading to emotional stability and constructive expression of thoughts and feelings.

Patanjali's eight limbs of yoga begin with *yama*, guidelines for social conduct, and *niyama*, guidelines for inner conduct. In fact, the yamas and niyamas do not belong only to raja yoga, but to all religions and spiritual paths of the world. In raja yoga there are five yamas and five niyamas, and in other systems there may be a few more. As already discussed in chapter 7, the yamas are *satya*, truthfulness, *ahimsa*, non-violence, *asteya*, honesty, *brahmacharya*, constant awareness of higher consciousness by restraining associations with sense experiences, and *aparigraha*, possessing only what is necessary. The niyamas are *shaucha*, cleanliness, *santosha*, contentment, *tapas*, austerities, *swadhyaya*, self-observation, and *Ishwara pranidhana*, surrendering to the will of higher consciousness. A process of inner transformation starts when we bring even one yama and one niyama into our lives. Emotional upheavals begin to settle down and life finds its direction. The mind becomes clear.

The modern sage Swami Sivananda, of Rishikesh has also presented an eight-limbed path of yoga. The eight steps of

Sivananda Yoga are serve, love, give, be good, do good, purify, meditate and realize. In essence it charts the path of the bhakti yoga concept that God is present in every living and non-living being, and to serve them is to serve God; to love them is to love God. The practice of serving humanity or other animals or planet Earth can also bring an end to personal suffering by changing the focus, and changing the karma and its fruit.

Writing a spiritual diary in order to observe oneself can be a very powerful practical way to deal with the emotions. The practices of bhakti yoga described earlier in the chapter are also beneficial.

Each one of the above practices is sufficient singly or in combination.

Other remedies: Aromatherapy suggests the use of lavender oil, rose oil and marjoram oil to name just a few. Bach flower remedies may be useful. Herbalists recommend the use of chamomile, hops, passion flower, valerian, kava, ginseng, ginkgo biloba and other herbal remedies. Music or massage also help to soothe the emotions.

General measures: Make sure you are well nourished, well hydrated and getting adequate peaceful sleep. Regular brisk walks, exercise or playing a game or two of your favourite sport will help to settle the emotions.

Financial concerns

Many people are able to attend to their jobs only intermittently or not at all because of their health status. This can drastically cut down their income. Their physical and mental state may not allow them to manage their investments, adding to the financial constraint. In some countries, conventional medical treatments can turn out to be very expensive. When a person is not covered by insurance, this can become a highly stressful situation. There may also be concern for the future financial state of family members after one's death, or when one is unable to earn any longer.

General measures: First and foremost allow the mind to relax and become calm. Then collect all the relevant information, using different resources. Assess the situation in depth. Make decisions after consulting family members and trusted friends. Gain their trust and support. Make practical plans for the future, making as many arrangements as possible, including organizing the necessary legal documents and explaining these clearly to the person whom you trust the most. Trust the Almighty to take over when and where your efforts cease.

Fig. 8.2: Management of Emotions

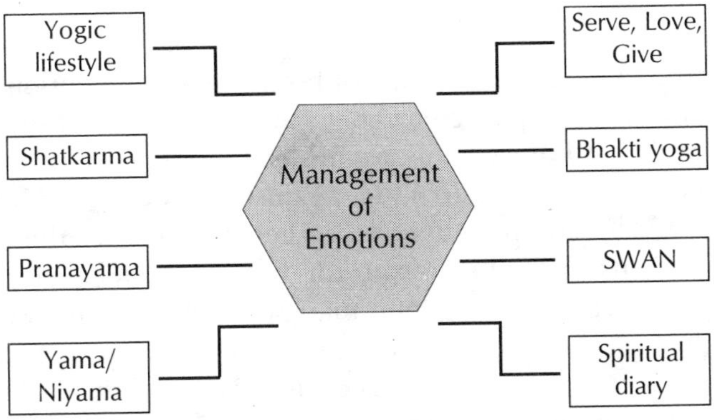

Note: The practices listed in this chapter are covered in the practice sections of previous chapters.

9

Eating Right

Diet is a very important part of both cancer prevention and therapy but no particular diet can be totally curative or preventive. All such claims are misleading. A good diet helps the body's resources to fight against cancer or any other disease. The components of the diet that protect the body from toxins are called protector nutrients. Beta-carotene, vitamin C, vitamin E, copper, manganese, selenium and zinc are thought to be protective. Mostly they act as antioxidants by removing free radicals. Free radicals are highly reactive, unstable molecules produced during the process of conversion of food into energy. Nutritional deficiencies may contribute to the genesis of cancer by suppressing the immune system and inducing premature ageing.

Dietary factors are believed to be responsible for about one-third of all cancers.[7] An appropriate diet creates an environment at the cellular and subtler mental level that is detrimental to the survival of the cancer cell. Healthy dietary habits help one to stay healthy, away from cancer and all other major diseases, but are no guarantee against ill health. There is no point becoming obsessive or worked up over dietary issues. One needs to take care in a relaxed, cautious manner.

In the following discussion an attempt is made to draw attention to the qualities of a healthy diet that promotes good health and in particular helps fight cancer.

Balanced diet

The metabolic rate of an individual depends on their age, gender, physical activity and endocrine status. If there is repeated consumption of more calories than the body needs, then weight is gained, whereas consuming too few calories over a period of time leads to weight loss. Normally the quantity of food eaten should be such that the body weight remains more or less constant and within the normal range. Obesity increases the risk of cancer and most other major diseases such as dyslipidemia, diabetes, hypertension, heart disease and arthritis, to name just a few. Similarly, people who are underweight and malnourished have weak immune systems and are more susceptible to infections and possibly to cancer.

The food we eat should be balanced in nutritive value. It should consist of 15–20% protein, 10–20% fat and the remaining 55–75% carbohydrate. In addition, it should contain all the vitamins and minerals that the body needs.

Carbohydrates are of two main types: simple carbohydrates such as are found in sugar, jaggery, honey and fruits, and complex carbohydrates such as are found in rice and other cereals, and pulses. Complex carbohydrates are preferable and should make up the major chunk of the carbohydrates we eat. The simple carbohydrates should only make up about 10% of the carbohydrate intake.

Proteins come from two sources, animal and plant. Animal proteins such as meat, chicken, fish, eggs, milk and milk products should be minimized and replaced by plant proteins as far as conveniently possible. Fish is the least harmful among the animal proteins. Overall plant proteins and fats are healthier for every adult than proteins and fats of animal origin. The cancer process by itself may or may not be directly related to animal proteins, and in fact if a person becomes very weak during the course of the disease, they may actually be recommended by the treating doctor. Fruits and vegetables definitely have a protective effect on many common cancers.[8]

Proteins are the building blocks of the body. Cancer cells consume the nutrients available in the blood, depriving normal cells of what they need. To prevent the malnourishment of normal cells, it is recommended that cancer patients include a good amount of protein in their diet. Proteins are more difficult to digest than carbohydrates, and the body uses more energy in digesting them. Proteins produce nitrogenous substances when they are broken down and these are eliminated from the body by the kidneys. A high protein diet is a load on both the digestive system and in some cases on the kidneys. A diet unduly rich in protein is not necessary and could be harmful. It is important to find the right balance.

Fat, like protein, comes from both animal and plant sources. Animal fat should be avoided as far as possible. Select lean meat or fat-free milk, for example. Excess fat in the diet is the most threatening dietary problem in the affluent world. Some forms of fat are more harmful than others. However, fat is an essential ingredient of our diet and total abstinence is not recommended. In terms of general health, an adult needs 10–15 ml of oil each day. Mustard oil, soy bean oil and safflower oil are preferable to peanut oil and sesame oil. Hydrogenated oil, butter and coconut oil should be avoided.

Salt or sodium and chloride ions are available in fruits and vegetables along with other minerals. Less than six grams of table salt a day is enough for any individual. A diet high in salt is harmful. Too much salt in the body places an extra workload on the kidneys, which are responsible for its excretion. Salt binds to water molecules and together they are retained in the body, which in certain circumstances may produce symptoms such as swelling, and a rise in blood pressure.

Sugar: Excessive consumption of sugar and other refined carbohydrates (such as refined flour) create favourable conditions for tumours to grow by lowering the oxygen level in the tissues. Sugar also stimulates the production of certain chemicals in the body which, when accumulated in large quantities, may in the long run further promote the growth of cancer.

Vitamins, minerals and antioxidants play an important role. It is best to include a wide variety of cereals, pulses, nuts, vegetables, roots and fruits in the diet. Consuming only one kind of cereal and a limited variety of fruits and vegetables is not desirable. No food article is complete by itself. Each cereal, pulse, vegetable or fruit is unique. Different trace elements (vitamins, minerals etc.) are found in different food articles.

One should try to include vegetables and fruits of different colours: green, such as spinach, broccoli, capsicum and grapes; yellow, such as potato, pumpkin, peaches, oranges, bananas and mangoes; red, such as tomatoes, carrots, beetroot, strawberries and plums; lightly coloured, such as cauliflower, cabbage, cucumber and melons. This will ensure the inclusion of necessary vitamins, minerals and trace elements as well as antioxidants.

Vegetarians can only obtain oil soluble vitamins from nuts, seeds and milk, and milk is their major source of calcium. Vegetables and fruits should be eaten fresh. Preserved food articles, including frozen food, lose many vital elements. When there is no alternative, frozen food is preferable to other types of preserved and processed foods. Citrus fruits, nuts, various sprouted seeds, and the juice of white gourds, carrots, aloe vera and wheat grass are said by some to particularly boost the body's own healing power.

Fibre content is also very important in the diet. Fibre is a complex carbohydrate. Being non-absorbable, it traps water and provides bulk to the waste content of the large intestine. It relieves constipation and keeps the digestive tract clean. It traps cholesterol and free oxygen radicals, thus preventing their absorption into the blood and body systems. In these ways, fibre contributes to the prevention of cancer and metabolic disorders such as hypertension and diabetes. The chief sources of fibre are fresh fruits with skin, whole grains, oatmeal, bran, and vegetables. The recommended minimum intake is 400 grams per day. The current view is that fruits and green and yellow vegetables are more important than fibre per se.

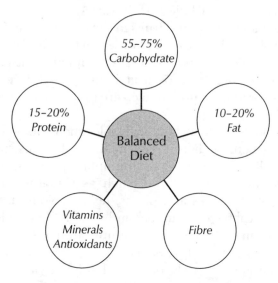

Fig. 9.1: A Balanced Diet

Raw foods: The diet should always include some raw, uncooked food such as sprouts, salad, fruit or juice, though too much raw food is not suitable for the human digestive system, which is not designed to handle large quantities of raw food. Raw vegetables or fruits are preferable to juices because the fibre and other contents are not wasted and the chewing muscles are exercised. The process of mastication (chewing) actually stimulates digestion. The digestion of carbohydrates is designed to begin in the mouth. Today people have developed the habit of consuming very soft and finely ground, easily gulp-able foodstuffs. Having said this, when a large quantity of a particular food is advised or is not chewable in its raw form, then the juice is recommended, for example, carrot juice and wheat grass juice.

Natural foods: The ingredients of the diet should be grown naturally without chemical fertilizers or pesticides. Some genetically manipulated hybrid varieties may not be safe. Agricultural produce that has undergone genetic engineering may also be harmful.

Alcohol: Some cancers have been linked to alcohol use. It is thought that alcohol may stimulate the growth of cancer by suppressing the activity of the natural killer cells (NK cells). It also directly harms normal cells. Alcoholic beverages should be avoided as much as possible because they affect the balance of the mind and also contribute to the development of a host of other disorders such as anxiety and stomach ulcers.

Some recommended foods[9]

Soya beans, sesame seeds, pistachios, walnuts and spinach contain *Co-enzyme Q10* in large quantities. Co-enzyme Q10 protects the liver, kidneys and heart from the damaging effects of free radicals.

Beta carotene, a precursor of vitamin A, increases the body's immunity against cancer by enhancing the activity of its NK cells. It is also an antioxidant. It helps protect the body against many cancers, including cancers of the cervix, lung and stomach. Most vegetables and yellow coloured fruits are rich in beta carotene. Carrots, sweet potatoes and spinach are particularly good sources.

Vitamin A also enhances the activity of the body's immune cells against cancer. It is found to be useful particularly in squamous cell carcinoma of the lungs, squamous cell carcinoma of the head and neck region, and malignant melanomas.

Vitamin B3 in a dose of 50 mg per day enhances the therapeutic effects of chemotherapy and radiotherapy. Asparagus, whole grains and brewer's yeast are rich sources of vitamin B3.

Vitamin B6 is found to be useful in protecting the respiratory tract from pollutants and infections, in cancers of the liver, cervix and bladder, and in the management of the side effects of radiotherapy. Bananas, apples, carrots, sweet potatoes and leafy green vegetables contain high quantities of vitamin B6.

Vitamin C enhances the immunity of the body by boosting the production of interferon and stimulating NK cells. It inhibits the growth of cancer by blocking the production of nitrosamines. Vitamin C also protects the body from the toxic side effects of chemotherapy and radiotherapy. It strengthens and stabilizes connective tissue around the tumour, thus inhibiting the spread of cancer. Vitamin C is found in many fruits and vegetables, including citrus fruits, broccoli and green peppers.

Vitamin D and its metabolites prevent the growth of cancer and induce the conversion of cancerous cells into normal cells. These effects have been studied in cancer of the prostate in particular.

Vitamin E, by its strong antioxidant effect, protects against chemical carcinogens. It reduces the toxic side effects of chemotherapy and radiotherapy. Dark green leafy vegetables, wheat grass and unrefined vegetable oils have a rich vitamin E content.

Folic acid plays an important role in the synthesis of DNA and protects the body against cancer, particularly cervical cancer. Cabbage, dark green leafy vegetables, citrus fruits and dairy products are high in folic acid.

Gamma linolenic acid inhibits the growth of cancer by producing PGE-1. It is promoted by vitamin B3, vitamin B6, vitamin C and zinc. Blackcurrant oil, evening primrose oil and mother's milk are rich sources of gamma linolenic acid.

Omega-3 fatty acids protect the body from cancer by inhibiting the production of harmful chemicals like PGE-2. They enhance the therapeutic effect of chemotherapy by altering the cell membranes of cancerous cells. They should only be taken in moderate quantities and always along with adequate amounts of antioxidants. They are known to protect the body against cancers of the breast and the liver. Fish, and plant oils such as flaxseed, pumpkin seed, corn, safflower, sunflower and walnuts are rich in omega-3 fatty acids.

The anti-cancer activity of *fibre* is due to its ability to eliminate toxins via the digestive tract. Legumes, cereals, grains, green vegetables and fruits, especially citrus fruits, are high in fibre.

Lactobacilli found in the human intestines protect the body against cancer by detoxifying chemical carcinogens. They produce the B group of vitamins which enhance the immunity of the body.

Zinc has an important role in the synthesis of DNA. It protects the body against all cancers, but particularly prostate cancer. Zinc is found in onions, grains, soybeans and sunflower seeds.

Selenium is a trace element essential in the detoxification process. It also enhances the activity of NK cells and arrests micro-metastases. It stimulates enzymes that repair DNA. Selenium is found to have a protective effect against all cancers, particularly those of the liver, leukaemia, colon, rectum, prostate, ovary, breast and lung. Some scientists recommend an intake of 200 mcg of selenium per day.

Iodine helps the body fight against cancer, especially breast cancer. Iodized salt and seaweeds provide good supplies of iodine.

Potassium helps to repair damaged DNA. High potassium and low sodium may help in reversing the process of carcinogenesis. Most fruits are rich in potassium. Coconut water is an extremely rich source of potassium.

Magnesium provides a protective effect against cancer by helping in the synthesis of DNA and maintaining the pH balance in body tissues. It is found in nuts, seafood, wheat-germ, bananas, grains, brown rice and green vegetables.

Calcium has a protective effect against cancer of the colon. It may be taken with magnesium to improve absorption. Nuts, dark green vegetables such as broccoli, and particularly milk, provide calcium in the diet.

Germanium is a trace element which inhibits cancerous growth by creating an oxygen rich environment around the cells. It also decreases the side effects of chemotherapy and radiotherapy.

Molybdenum, a trace element, protects the body, especially against cancer of the oesophagus.

Chromium helps in the synthesis of glucose tolerance factor. Prolonged consumption of refined carbohydrates such as sugar and white flour (which are extremely poor in chromium) may lead to hyperglycaemia, which promotes the synthesis of harmful chemicals like PGE-2, leading to carcinogenesis.

Manganese is a co-factor in the synthesis of many enzymes, including antioxidants. It also counteracts the immuno-suppressive effects of the hormone cortisone released during stressful periods.

Table 9.1: Source of Important Food Nutrients

Food Nutrient	Found in
Co-enzyme Q10	*Soya beans, sesame seeds, pistachios, walnuts, spinach*
Beta carotene	*Vegetables, especially carrots, sweet potatoes and spinach, and yellow coloured fruits*
Vitamin B3	*Asparagus, whole grains, brewer's yeast*
Vitamin B6	*Bananas, apples, carrots, sweet potatoes, leafy green vegetables*
Vitamin C	*Citrus fruits, broccoli, green pepper*
Vitamin E	*Dark green leafy vegetables, wheat grass, unrefined vegetable oils*
Folic acid	*Cabbage, dark green leafy vegetables, citrus fruits, dairy products*
Omega–3 fatty acids	*Fish, walnuts, plant oils such as flaxseed, pumpkin seed, corn, safflower and sunflower*
Fibre	*Legumes, cereals, grains, green vegetables, fruits, especially citrus*
Zinc	*Onions, grains, soybeans, sunflower seeds*
Potassium	*Coconut water, fruits*
Iodine	*Seaweeds, iodized salt*
Magnesium	*Nuts, seaweed, wheatgerm, bananas, grains, brown rice, green vegetables*
Calcium	*Nuts, dark green vegetables like broccoli, milk*

Preparation of food

The way in which food is prepared is very important. The correct method of preparation preserves the *prana* or vitality in the food. The ancient way of cooking very slowly on a low fire helps to preserve the vitality of food. Overcooked food loses its vitality and undercooked food is difficult to digest. High temperature fast cooking, charcoal smoking, barbecuing, deep frying, microwave cooking and pressurized cooking are not healthy ways of preparing food. Of these, pressurized cooking is the least harmful. The water used for simmering food should not be thrown out as it contains vital nutrients. Food should be prepared only a little prior to eating. Fruits and vegetables should not be cut up too long before the actual cooking or eating time. Similarly, juices should be freshly squeezed. The right kind of spices and condiments can enhance the quality or reduce a side effect of a particular food item. They can also help bring out the taste and enhance the digestive capacity.

The *frame of mind* at the time of preparing food can affect the properties of the food. The emotions of the person cooking the food are carried into that food. A happy person, cooking with love and good wishes for those who are going to eat, adds a lot of vitality to food. Similarly, an angry or depressed person steals the vitality from the food while cooking. At the time of cooking think that you are cooking for your most beloved one or your Lord. This food is going to bring the feeling of total satisfaction to the people who consume it and nourish them at all levels. It is a medium for expressing your love and a vehicle for the divine grace to flow to other people. Our mothers and grandmothers used to chant the Lord's name or sing beautiful songs while working in the kitchen.

The way to eat

Food must be fully respected. In the ancient Indian culture food was considered as *prasad*, the grace of God. Life was considered to be a *yajna*, a sacred ceremony. In the yajna of life an action for the benefit of society is offered as a sacrifice and God, or

247

the higher force, gives food (and other personal benefits) as His grace. Food is eaten not for enjoyment, but as an *offering to the inner fire* to keep it burning. This inner fire is the store-house of *prana*, energy. The following verse from the *Bhagavad Gita* (4:24), often chanted before a meal, conveys this idea.

ब्रह्मार्पणंऽब्रह्मऽहविर्ब्रह्माग्नौऽब्रह्मणाहुतम्ऽ ।
ब्रह्मैवऽतेनऽगन्तव्यंऽब्रह्मकर्मसमाधिनाऽ ॥

Brahmaarpanam brahma havirbrahmaagnau brahmanaahutam
Brahmaiva tena gantavyam brahmakarmasamaadhinaa

Brahman (cosmic energy) is the oblation; Brahman is the clarified butter etc. constituting the offerings; Brahman pours the oblation into the fire of Brahman; Brahman verily shall be reached by him who always sees Brahman in all actions.

In many other cultures, grace or a prayer of thanksgiving is said before eating. It is best to eat in a relaxed and happy mood. When a meal is eaten in a hurry, it may provide calories but not vitality. When the mind is agitated at the time of eating, the food cannot be digested and can turn into poison. Unpleasant emotions are a very powerful destructive force and can vitiate the food in the digestive system. It is wiser to delay the meal until the mind settles down. The ritual of offering food as thanksgiving – to one's personal god, to the fire for allowing the cooking to happen, to guests and renunciates as a token of respect, to dependents, poor people and animals and birds – as a token of love has deep significance. It is an effective way to prepare the mind for the act of eating. It converts the act of eating into an act of worship. Other considerations are a pleasant dining area, a shower before a meal, gentle music and so on.

According to Ayurveda, food should be eaten only when there is a desire to eat. Maintaining regular mealtimes is a health promoting habit. It helps the biological clock to set itself and the digestive glands to work more efficiently. Yoga advocates eating when the breath is flowing more easily through the right nostril. Food should be chewed sufficiently. It is said that solid food should be drunk and liquids should be eaten. This means that solid food should be chewed so much that by being mixed with saliva, it becomes a liquid that can be drunk, and that liquids must be taken slowly as if it is solid food that is being swallowed.

In relation to how much to eat at a meal, it is recommended that the stomach should be half filled with solid food, a quarter with liquid and the remaining quarter kept empty. Eating to full capacity and overeating invite ill health. At the time of eating, the awareness should be focused on food and the process of eating; other business can be put aside for a while. After finishing the meal, sitting peacefully for few moments is a good habit. Yoga recommends sitting in vajrasana, or doing *vamakukshi*, lying on left side for about ten minutes watching the breath and the movements of the abdomen. Heavy physical activity should be postponed for one to two hours.

Other miscellaneous things to avoid

Bitter tasting cereals, peanuts and corn may contain aflatoxins, a carcinogen caused by mould. Consumption of milk from cows treated with bovine growth hormone may contribute to cancer genesis.

In summary

The World Health Organization says, "A diet that is low in total and saturated fats, high in plant foods, especially green and yellow vegetables and fruits, low in alcohol, low in salt-pickled, smoked and salt-preserved foods is consistent with a low risk of many of the current major cancers, cardiovascular diseases, obesity, diabetes and many other diseases."[10]

Recommendations from a yogic viewpoint include an easily digestible, high fibre, vegetarian, balanced diet, cooked properly and eaten at the proper time, in moderation, while in a positive frame of mind. This is a strong weapon in the fight against cancer and ill health.

10

Beyond Cancer with Yoga

After undergoing the ordeal of cancer, from first hearing the diagnosis to the various treatment regimes with their side effects, when the medical reports start becoming normal, it can feel like being born again or being given a boon of new life. It is like a plant surviving through a hurricane storm due to its strong root system (inner strength), supported by the firmness of the soil and the help of neighbouring plants (family, friends and health system) in helping to break the force of the storm to some extent. Now, the sun is seen rising over the horizon.

After every storm the sky becomes clearer and visibility is enhanced and sharpened. In the same way, after the cancer is eradicated and one has been through the life-changing experience of dealing with it, the perspectives on life can become clearer. One should take best possible advantage of this opportunity and not let it slip away.

With the help of yoga, a great deal can be achieved in the following areas:
- Continuing to strengthen the body and improve overall health.
- Considering one's present needs, at all levels, and finding ways to meet them.
- Discovering the purpose of life, and working towards it.
- Emotions and relationships.

It can be very helpful to continue to pay attention to the area of emotions and relationships. When passing through challenging situations, it can be very easy to develop low self-esteem, due to over-emphasizing the individual limitations that become exposed. Unfulfilled expectations may also give rise to bitterness, affecting relationships. Relationships with others can be improved by appreciating every little piece of help that is offered, and then spreading the naturally arising feelings of benevolence and sense of duty towards our fellow human beings: those close to us and those we do not know. After successful treatment, it is natural for the fear of recurrence of cancer to lurk in the mind, at the conscious and subconscious levels. Similarly, the experience of cancer makes the fear of death alive and real. These fears need to be attended to. The practices of yoga aid the continued work on emotions and thought patterns that obstruct our growth and expansion of consciousness, and limit our positive experience and expression in life.

It is important to continue with the practice of yoga that connects one with one's own inner core, and through that, to others and the cosmic energy or the divine. The three areas of yogic practices, positive attitudes and yogic lifestyle have already been discussed and practised. When the appropriate practices and attitudes (asana, pranayama, yoga nidra, dharana practices such as ajapa japa, mantra japa, mantra meditation and sadbhavana meditation, yama and niyama, SWAN practice and spiritual diary) are incorporated into a yogic lifestyle, the sun of health and happiness can shine throughout life.

An account by a yoga practitioner who used the practices of yoga, especially yoga nidra, to heal herself from cancer, showing that yoga can be used not only to help recover and heal from cancer, but also after this process, to live in a better way, is included as an Appendix.

251

11

Fear of Death

When a diagnosis of cancer is first heard, instantaneously one thinks of suffering and death – frightening thoughts. But to die, a person needs no disease. When the time is up, one dies with disease or without, regardless of full health and vigour. Like a ripened fruit falling off a tree of its own accord, everyone passes away when the call comes from the inner clock.

Drs Kothari and Mehta[11] narrate a beautiful verse by G. K. Chesterton.

> *Six detectives went fishing*
> *Down by the seaside.*
> *They found a dead body*
> *And inquired how it died.*
> *Father Brown informed them*
> *Quite mild and without scorn:*
> *'Like you and me and the rest of us,*
> *He died of being born.'*

Fear of death is a basic instinct. We are all born with it. No one wants to die. Any creature, big or small, will try its best to escape the extinction of its life. Sage Patanjali in the *Yoga Sutras* calls this fear of death *abhinivesha*. He describes it as the last of the five fundamental tendencies or characteristics of the human mind.

Causes of fear

There are many reasons for a fear of death. The first one is the sense of losing life, losing everything that is familiar to us: our family, our home, the work we are used to doing, our possessions, even our name and identity. The second reason is fear of the unknown, the realization that we are about to enter into an unknown, totally unfamiliar realm. The third reason is the anticipation of suffering and unpleasantness, dependence on others and losing our dignity due to physical incapacity during terminal illness.

However, if we knew that in losing everything that is familiar to us, we would be gaining something very precious and beautiful, we would not be afraid of death. If we knew that we were returning to our original home, we would not be afraid. If we were convinced that the soul, the real us, does not suffer or feel humiliated, we would not be afraid. In this day and age we are also very fortunate that our physical sufferings and incapacities can be well managed with the help of modern facilities. The release from the physical and subsequent subtler bodies can be experienced in meditation or spiritual practices, and in this way we can become familiar with the process. Through this, we become convinced that life does not depend only on functioning through the physical body, and that beyond the body there is more freedom and expansion of consciousness. Fear of death and the unknown beyond death can then be fully overcome.

Teachings from the Upanishads also tell us that death is not a fearful or horrifying event. It is an essential phase of life and has to be accepted like other occasions. In earlier parts of the Vedas, the lord of death is considered to be a guide who takes people to the doors of heaven! But in the later period, death assumed a ferocious and threatening outlook and became the lord of bereavement. With the passage of time, vices crept into society and it was deemed necessary to warn people away from evils, and for this purpose the horrifying concept of hell and the god of death evolved.

The theory of rebirth

Eastern philosophies believe that the spirit or soul is eternal. When it comes to planet Earth it wears the garb of the physical body and functions through it. After undergoing various experiences it leaves the body and its existence on planet Earth and travels to other realms of existence where it assimilates the learning into knowledge. It then plans the area of further experiences needed and chooses the next birth accordingly. Its past karmas and state of mind at the time of death give a direction to its next birth. It comes back again and again until it realizes its true nature, which is the same as the Cosmic Self. When it acquires this ultimate knowledge, it becomes liberated from the cycles of birth and death and merges into the Cosmic Self.

According to the theory of rebirth, the same soul, atman, keeps coming back to planet Earth in the vehicles of different bodies. So though there is loss of function and breath in that body, the soul again starts functioning and breathing in yet another body. It has the capacity to revive its memory of all the previous births, and it has the capacity to stay conscious, not only in the state of consciousness, but also in the states of dream, sleep, death and after-death, because the soul remains the same throughout different states of the body.

This theory is illustrated in the following verses from the *Bhagavad Gita*.

It (the soul) is never born nor does it ever die; after having been, it again ceases not to be. It is without birth, eternal, changeless and ancient. It is not destroyed when the body is destroyed. (2:20)

Just as in this body the embodied (soul) passes into childhood, youth and old age, so also does he pass into another body; the wise person does not grieve at it. (2:13)

Just as a person discards an old garment and puts on a new one, similarly the occupant of the body (the soul) discards the old incapable body and enters a new one. (2:22)

Everything that is born must perish one day, and after destruction, it is sure to obtain a new life. Therefore, it is not worth grieving over something that is inevitable.

(2:27)

The theory of rebirth is supported by many spiritual systems. Vedic Dharma, popularly known as Hinduism, is its main source. Buddhism and Jainism also believe in it. It is said that even the Christian Church, no doubt under the influence of eastern philosophies, held to the doctrine of rebirth until the middle of the sixth century. In the year 553 AD the doctrine was rejected by the Second Council of Constantinople, with one third of the bishops present voting for the retention of the doctrine and the rest voting against.

Some spiritual systems do not support the theory of rebirth. However, all believe that the soul is an extension of the Cosmic Self – that after death it returns to higher realms and at an appropriate time merges with the Cosmic Self. In short, death is a characteristic of the physical body, not of the soul. Our essential self is a part of the immortal and always stays immortal.

Beings are experienced to be unmanifest in their beginning, are seen to be manifest in their middle state and are noticed to be unmanifest again in their end. What is there then to grieve about? (*Bhagavad Gita*, 2:28)

Choice of next birth

The emotional state of the mind and the level of awareness at the time of death are decided by the way one has lived one's life. If wealth was the driving force behind one's activities, then one would tend to think or worry about wealth; if, on the other hand, the family was the point of attraction, then the mind would revolve around that at the time of death. The strongest thought (desire) at the time of death decides the next type of birth.

Whosoever at the end leaves the body, thinking of any being, to that being only does he go because of his constant thought of that being. *(Bhagavad Gita, 8:6)*

Our past karmas also guide the direction that our next life will take. If we have lived a good life, fulfilled our duties sincerely and tried to improve our qualities, we will be born into a good family and will continue to grow spiritually.

PERSPECTIVES ON DEATH

Death is a celebration

Death is a beautiful event if we have the capacity to experience it correctly. Osho describes death as an event of festivity, joy and celebration. All the saints of the world have unanimously proclaimed life as suffering and death as an opportunity to experience bliss. There may be physical suffering due to the presence of a disease, but it can be taken care of by medical or other therapeutic intervention. If the mind can be kept dissociated from the happenings in the body, in a cheerful mood, the process of actual dying is very blissful and can take one to the heights of ecstasy. The key is to link with the Cosmic Self through linking with the individual soul. A lifetime of practising meditation is a very good preparation for this crucial and precious moment. One who has lived life simply and with childlike innocence and purity can spontaneously form this link without any prior experience in meditation.

According to vedic scriptures, death is suffused in light. Immortality is reached only through death. No one becomes immortal with the body. Death is not evil. It leads man to the world of God and God to the world of man.

People today concentrate on life and tend to avoid and even deny all dealings with the dying and the dead. This attitude is fundamentally different from traditional thought in which both birth and death are held as occasions for celebration.

Death is a time for learning

Dying is a time for growth and achievement. Just as bedtime is the time to reflect upon the day's activities and the year's end is the time to settle one's accounts, dying is the time to reflect over the life's events as a spectator. It is the best opportunity to understand oneself and to grow.

Annie Besant writes[12]: "The casting off of the physical body is termed death in the ordinary sense. The etheric double or pranic body consisting of automatic vitality (link between individual prana and cosmic prana) and energizing vitality (individual prana) leaves the physical body and hovers around the physical body in the form of a hazy translucent body very similar to the physical body. As long as its connection with the physical body is maintained, the body can be revived to life again. While it is still connected to the body, it relives the experiences of the whole life again and sums up the learning of that life. It reads its life remaining as a spectator. This is a moment of great spiritual learning. An atmosphere of peace, love and honour for the dying person facilitates this process. An atmosphere of violent emotions or emotionally holding on to the dying person creates obstacles in the journey ahead. In a few seconds to many minutes the connection becomes severed and the pranic body is cast off on the earth plane side by side with the physical body."

Death is a spiritual experience

Death is a highly charged spiritual state wherein one can transcend the usual conditionings of the mind, expand beyond the limitations of the 'I-mine' concept with minimum effort and establish a link with the higher energy. People who have had a near death experience (NDE) stand witness to this.

Death is delightful and friendly. What is considered anecdotal is in fact a fairly common illuminating death experience, bordering on the divine or the supernatural. Regardless of age, sex, past illness, past deeds, learnedness or otherwise, the act of dying bestows on an individual a beautiful and blissful experience, devoid of any sense of fear, with unseen loving guides close enough not to allow the dying person to feel lonely. Before breathing their last, dying persons move away from their physical self to serve as witness to the event. Dying persons who have returned to life 'from the embrace of eternity' stress the need in this life of cultivating love for others as the prime necessity of existence.

Melvin Morse and Paul Perry[13] say that the experience is not frightening at all. All the pain and suffering disappear. One thing common to all those who have experienced NDE is a feeling of peace, divinity and bliss. Many people later say that they know they can die at any time and yet have no fear of death. The experience is superimposed upon the experience of the reality that is actually going on at the deathbed. One or more of the following are experienced during a NDE:

1. Being out of the physical body
2. Travelling up a sort of tunnel
3. Seeing a light, usually very luminous but gentle and reassuring or comforting
4. Visiting known or unknown people who are dead
5. Seeing a being of light
6. Having a life review
7. Deciding to return to the physical body.

Pre-death visions have many things in common with NDE. The dying person may find relief in pain and other discomforts, may have visions of other worlds and conversations with dead loved ones. The dying person perceives that the departed loved ones have come to take him away.

Not only the person who is dying, but also everyone around them come under this spell of spirituality.

To summarize, most of the fears woven around death can be managed very successfully by accepting the inevitability of death, letting go of the old conditionings of the mind and by planning and executing accordingly the affairs of our life and of the people around us.

YOGA NIDRA

Experiencing the subtle body

Please start the practice with the first four stages of yoga nidra (preparation and relaxation, resolve, rotation of consciousness and breathing. Stage 5 (feelings and sensations) may be omitted. Then continue with one of the following visualization alternatives.

Stage 6: Visualization

1. **Floating body**: Imagine that you are on the ceiling . . . and you see below you your body lying in shavasana on the floor, practising yoga nidra beside other people. *(pause)* Now see your body slowly stand up and tiptoe to the door, quietly open it . . . and go outside, closing the door softly behind you. See your body walking outside this building, see the familiar things around you . . . there is no sense of effort, only lightness. *(pause)* You meet some people that you know . . . see them, but they can't see you. Watch them as they walk past, perhaps they are making their usual conversation. *(pause)* Suddenly you find that your body is floating over the sea . . . become aware of this . . . see the dark blue sea glistening below, across its surface a ship is steaming. *(pause)* Your body floats like a cloud . . . wherever the wind blows the clouds, your body is also blown . . . wisps of cloud brush past your face. Below you sunlight reflects off banks of white cloud . . . above you puffs of

cloud scurry across a blue sky. *(pause)* Now your body is lifted by currents of air and carried over the land . . . on the ground below you see farmhouses, carefully laid out fields, thick forests, winding rivers that reflect the sun. *(pause)* Pause a moment and look closely at yourself . . . your body is totally relaxed and on your face is an expression of peace and calm. *(pause)* See your body suddenly immersed in colour as it passes through a rainbow . . . feel yourself washed and purified by subtle colours . . . yellow, green, blue, violet, red, orange, golden yellow. Feel the colours penetrating your whole body, nourishing and invigorating you at some deep level. *(long pause)* Then slowly make your return . . . see your body return to the outside of this building . . . see again the familiar objects. Quietly open the door, walk inside and close it after you. You lie down on the floor, taking care not to disturb other people. *(pause)* Now see your body slowly practising some asanas . . . your body rests again in shavasana. *(long pause)* Now repeat your resolve three times mentally with full conviction.

2. **Tunnel of chidakasha**: Withdraw your mind and concentrate on the space in front of the forehead. It is called chidakasha. Do not strain your eyes at all. Let all the eye muscles stay relaxed. *(pause)* Watch the darkness carefully, but without involvement. Feel at home in this warm and friendly darkness. *(pause)* Now start exploring the space of chidakasha. Try to find its floor. *(pause)* It is bottomless. There is no floor. Try to find its roof. *(pause)* You cannot find any ceiling or roof. Explore the right and then the left boundaries. *(pause)* No walls can be found on either right or left side. Allow your awareness to travel in front and then back. *(pause)* No limits can be found. The dark space is limitless. It is infinite. *(pause)* As you are exploring the space you find a faint light coming from nowhere. Try to reach that light. *(pause)* While tracing the source of the light, find yourself entering a tunnel. You are travelling

up the tunnel smoothly, effortlessly and safely. You have no fear. It is a very peaceful and pleasant experience. As you are travelling ahead the light is getting brighter and clearer. *(pause)* Now you are out of the tunnel. You are bathing in, floating in, this gentle, caressing, nurturing luminosity. *(pause)* It is a divine experience, most fulfilling and blissful. *(pause)* Now gradually allow the luminosity to become dim and be extinguished. *(pause)* Become aware of the dark space of chidakasha. *(pause)* Now repeat your resolve or sankalpa three times mentally with full conviction. *(pause)*

Stage 8: Ending the practice

Become aware of your body. *Pause.* Become aware of your natural breath.

Gradually externalize the mind and the senses. Begin moving the different parts of the body.

Note: The 'tunnel of chidakasha' visualization can also be done as a dharana practice. In that case it is preceded by the practice of kaya sthairyam as given in the practice section for chapter 5.

12

Preparation for Dying

Nothing in life is to be feared. It is only to be understood well and after understanding it, an appropriate action taken. This principle also holds true in the case of death. We need to understand that death is inevitable and that it can grasp only the physical body. We need to understand that the inner essential self is beyond the clutches of death and that death is a blissful experience of the individual self coming closer to or merging into the Cosmic Self. Our excessive involvement in 'I-and-my' can create obstacles to this blissful experience. We also need to be accustomed to the process of connecting to the inner self and the Cosmic Self. So we need to prepare and rehearse for this important event of life. Lack of preparation and attachment to 'I-mine' are the causes of pain experienced at the time of death.

Living well is dying well
The first point in preparation for dying in a good manner is living in a good manner. A life lived in harmony with oneself, with other beings and nature is a life well lived. We need to be considerate to plant life and wildlife as well. And we need to show the utmost consideration towards our fellow human beings. It is never too late. We can start now.

Those who can't live well can't die well, for dying is the last act that the living being performs. Living well is preserving the image of eternity, with which each person is born, undistorted and undisturbed. A genuine sense of reverence for the elements within and around us can help each one of us steer our life towards good living. Everything that throbs with life is an integral and interconnected part of the universe. Plant and animal life may be sacrificed to meet human necessities, but not for luxuries. The principles of a yogic lifestyle lead us to good living. Also, the yamas and niyamas can be very useful tools in our attempts at living well. We have already discussed yogic lifestyle as well as the yamas and niyamas in chapter 6.

This point of living well is also illuminated in the eight steps of Swami Sivananda's yoga, which are complementary to Patanjali's eight steps of yoga. In Patanjali's yoga the effort is to understand and improve the individual self. In Sivananda Yoga the effort is to recognize that one is a part of humanity, expressing one's best qualities. The eight steps are 'Serve, Love, Give, Purify, Be good, Do good, Meditate, Realize'. Service begins by connecting with other people, being able to put oneself in the shoes of the other person, being able to experience the suffering of the sufferer, and then not becoming a reformer, but using one's wisdom and attainments to find a way to help that person grow. As one starts thinking about others and helping others a beautiful quality develops within, known as love. Love is not the fulfilment of personal expectations. Real love is the ability to understand, appreciate and be one with the other person. In real love one feels for that person as one feels for oneself.

The third component is giving. When one learns to love, then there is no holding back; it is giving, giving and giving, without desiring anything in return. Giving is an art, the purpose of which is to help the recipient become independent and free. This leads to natural and spontaneous purification of the limiting tendencies of human nature. This purification does not mean an absence of negative qualities, but a state of wholeness and satisfaction where negative circumstances are unable to influence us. The next four components flow on naturally in a person who has adhered to the first four components. One need not be rich, strong or able in order to practise 'serve, love, give and purify'. Even a penniless, weak and sick, not so intelligent or homebound person can observe these principles in their daily dealings.

When the dying person is satisfied with their contribution and the attainments of their lifespan, and there are no more desires left to be fulfilled, then there is a joyous feeling even at the time of death.

Meditation

The second point in preparation is meditation practices. The practices of meditation help us to find and acquaint ourselves with our inner self. They help us to identify the universal link that connects all of us. They expand and fine-tune our consciousness beyond the realm of the conscious mind. Regular practice of meditation makes us ready to reap the maximum benefit of the unique spiritual experience at the time of death.

Often a mantra is used in meditation. Mantra is a syllable or word or a set of words. When the mantra is remembered consciously, it is automatically stored in the unconscious mind. At the time of parting, the mantra which is stored in the unconscious mind becomes one's guide. This period of separation is painful for the spiritually ignorant but not for the spiritual person who has remembered the mantra faithfully. The mantra serves as a guide through this period of transition. Mantra is a spiritual guide that dispels the fear of death and leads one fearlessly to the other shore of life.

AT THE TIME OF DYING

Surroundings at the time of dying

Peaceful, neat, clean and holy surroundings are preferable. An emotionally charged atmosphere of sorrow, pity, holding on to the person who is departing or disputes over family matters are not desirable. People should be very sensitive to

264

the needs of the person who is dying. Their heart should be full of love and respect for the departing soul. Light, incense, flowers, chanting of mantras or holy words or prayers, especially ones that are familiar to the departing person, and comforting and reassuring words and touch from the loved ones help very much.

At the time of dying

It is important to accept death wholeheartedly when it becomes imminent and be prepared adequately. As long as consciousness is maintained, stay connected with the spirit and the Lord within.

> If the embodied one meets death when sattwa is predominant, then he attains the stainless worlds of the knowers of the Highest. Meeting death in rajas, he is born among those attached to action; and dying in tamas, he is born in the womb of the senseless.
>
> *(Bhagavad Gita* (14:14–15)

The dying person should wind up his worldly affairs as much as possible. He should then withdraw his mind from the people and happenings of the external world and be engrossed in his meditative practice. If the mind becomes distracted, then bring it back again to the practice. Different spiritual systems have recommended various technically different but basically similar meditative practices for the occasion of dying. In essence, the awareness is gathered on one point (usually the heart centre or eyebrow centre) using mantra and symbol. With the power of this focused consciousness, the circulating prana or energy is gradually withdrawn from the peripheral parts of the body to central areas, and then from the lower end of the vertebral column to the eyebrow centre or the crown of head. Maintaining awareness of the mantra and symbol, consciousness is then allowed to escape from the body.

During life one needs to become accustomed to the practice of meditation to the stage of one-pointed concentration on the mantra and the symbol. When death is near, the natural process helps one to withdraw the prana and consciousness and allow them to escape from the body.

Meditations at the time of death

1. From *Bhagavata Mahapurana* (2.1.15–39):

Do not be afraid of death. Slay the attachment to the body and people related to the body with the weapon of *vairagya*, dispassion. Cleanse the body. Sit in a meditative asana in a clean, auspicious and solitary place. Begin mental japa of the mantra *Om*. Withdraw the senses from sense objects *(pratyahara)*. Withdraw the desire induced dissipated mind from its inner dialogue by conscious thinking *(antar mouna)*. Maintain awareness of *Om* chanting throughout. When the mind becomes quiet, attach it to the auspicious form of the Lord. Take the awareness to each and every part of the Lord's form one by one. When the mind becomes absolutely steady on one part, only then is it moved on to the next one. Let the mind be steady. If it wanders or drifts into slumber, patiently bring it back on to the form. Let the mind merge into the form of the Lord.

Then press the heel on the anus and direct the prana upwards, piercing the six chakras one by one. After reaching vishuddhi chakra, block the seven gates: the two eyes, two ears, two nasal openings and mouth, and direct the prana to ajna chakra. Stay there for a few minutes and then direct it to sahasrara. There merge the consciousness into Paramatma, the Cosmic Self, and allow the prana to leave through the *brahmarandhra* or fontanelle, leaving the mortal body behind.

2. From *Bhagavad Gita*: It is essentially the same as in *Bhagavata Mahapurana*.

Having closed all the gates (establishing pratyahara), having confined the mind in the heart, having fixed the life-breath in the 'head', engaged in the practice of concentration, uttering the one-syllabled Om, the (symbol of) Brahman and remembering Me, he who departs, leaving the body, attains the Supreme Goal.   (8:12–13)

At the time of death, with an unshaken mind full of devotion, by the power of yoga, fixing the whole prana (breath) in the middle of the two eyebrows, he reaches that supreme, resplendent Purusha.   (8:10)

And whosoever, leaving the body, goes forth remembering Me alone, at the time of death, attains My being; there is no doubt about this.   (8:5)

3. From *Ishavasya Upanishad* (v. 15–18): The last four verses of the *Ishavasya Upanishad* are well known as a prayer for the dying. These verses are worthy of being a prayer for the living as well.

A person who is dying experiences a very bright light, almost blinding, as he is preparing for the onward journey. He then prays to the light deity, the Sun. "The face of Brahman (ultimate Truth) is covered with golden light. O Pushan, O Nourisher, uncover this veil for me, who practises Truth or meditates on Truth, so that I may see Thee. The light is blinding me, disperse the rays and gather this light that is covering everything, so that I can see beyond the light."
At this point suddenly he beholds the vision of a supremely beautiful and auspicious divine form and acquires the self-realization that "I am Purusha, the all-pervading eternal being; Soham, I am That (Brahman)." He says, "Let my prana merge into the all-pervading air, and let my body be turned into ashes." He tells his mind to remember all his deeds, to review the whole of his life. It is an instantaneous insight into his whole life at the moment of death. He offers his salutations and requests Agni, the lord of fire, the knower of all paths, to lead him by a good path in his onward journey and to remove all the crooked sins from within him.

At the moment of death, a realization of one's true being has to take place, and this is the discovery of one's identity with the Divine Being (Purusha), whose vision is most glorious, beautiful and saving. It is a vision leading to this identification. Once this ultimate experience takes place, what remains of a person is the body, which returns to the earth element in the form of ashes, and his breath, which merges into the universal and immortal wind. What remains is also his karma, which can be burnt up in the very act of recollecting it, since the true identity is already discovered.

Appendix

Yoga Nidra: A Healing Practice for People Living with Cancer*

Julie Friedeberger (UK)

I have practised yoga nidra since 1985, and have been teaching it almost as long. In 1993, when I was diagnosed with breast cancer, yoga nidra became a central, indispensable part of my yoga practice, which as a whole was the key factor in my recovery, and in the longer term, my healing. This experience left me with a deeper trust in yoga and a stronger commitment to teaching it. Since then, the focus of my teaching has increasingly been on the healing power of yoga, and the ways in which the yoga practices can support the healing process.

Yoga and healing

The benefits of yoga nidra to general health and wellbeing, and its deeper spiritual effects, are known to everyone who practises it, and are doubly applicable to anyone confronting and living with a life-changing illness. In this article I offer my thoughts on the importance of yoga nidra for people who are living with cancer (or indeed any life-changing illness) and on the specific relevance for them of the individual components of the practice.

---

* Printed in *YOGA*, April 2008, Sivananda Math, Munger, India

I believe that the need for healing, for wholeness, harmony and balance is common to all beings; and that yoga and healing are fundamentally the same. These two beliefs are the foundation on which I base my teaching. The word 'yoga' means union: yoking, uniting, bringing together. The *Oxford Dictionary* defines the word 'heal' as: "To make whole, or sound; to unite, after being cut or broken." So yoga and healing share both meaning and goal: integration, harmony, and balance on all levels of our being; and at the deepest level, the uniting of the self with the Self. Yoga is holistic: it heals by making us whole.

We all need, and seek, healing. When a person faces a diagnosis of cancer, this need becomes urgent. Cancer pulls one into the present; it turns one's life inside out, demanding that every aspect of it be urgently examined and reassessed. The diagnosis can leave one feeling fragmented: people say "I felt as though I was in pieces," "I felt as though I had lost myself." This is an extremely intense experience, and it draws many who are searching for healing and the restoration of their wholeness to yoga.

Every aspect of yoga has a role to play in the healing process. Nurturing body movement, breathing exercises, meditation, relaxation, yoga nidra – all encourage the conditions in which physical, emotional, mental and spiritual health can flourish. Our efforts to observe yama and niyama give us the inner strength, conviction and faith to meet the challenges we face and to learn the lessons they hold for us. The sacred texts – the *Bhagavad Gita*, the Upanishads, Patanjali – guide and support our quest for knowledge and help us prepare for death. Perhaps most importantly, they show us that we can heal into death.

Relaxation

Relaxation is fundamental to healing. Bringing body and mind to rest encourages our inner healing forces to work for us, and any deep relaxation technique will have positive effects on health and wellbeing. Regularly practised, relaxation calms the sympathetic nervous system (which initiates the 'fight or flight' response) and activates the parasympathetic nervous system (which gives the message to body and mind that 'all is well'). Deep relaxation slows and regulates breathing, lowers heart rate and blood pressure, and releases muscular, mental and emotional tension. It improves one's quality of sleep and powers of concentration. It alleviates the anxiety and stress that depress immune function, and creates the conditions that enhance it. Since cancer, broadly speaking, is a complex of conditions in which a compromised immune system is failing to cope with the proliferation of damaged cells, a practice that stimulates the immune response is likely to be helpful.

Yoga nidra

Yoga nidra is a transformative practice that can bring about change on a profound level. Swami Satyananda Saraswati says: "The profound experience of muscular, mental and emotional relaxation attainable in yoga nidra enables a balance of psychic and vital energies within the psychic channels (*nadis*) of the energy framework underlying the physical body. Free flow of these energies forms the basis of optimal physical and mental health."[1]

To the general benefits of relaxation, yoga nidra adds special attributes of its own. It helps us to overcome fears, anxieties and insecurities. It creates an inner environment conducive to the transformation of attitudes. It teaches us to let go. It develops detachment (*vairagya*). It releases our samskaras. It awakens *sakshi*, the witnessing consciousness.

These will be the effects of yoga nidra for those who regularly practise it. For anyone dealing with a life-changing disease – and here we are not concerned solely with physical recovery, but with full emotional and spiritual healing – all these attributes become even more important and more necessary.

Every part of the practice of yoga nidra works to free blocked energy. Most significantly, practising yoga nidra can help us to acknowledge and accept the reality of our situation, however unwelcome, difficult, or scary it is; and can help us to acknowledge, accept, and release the powerful emotions it brings up. These emotions are understandably often bottled up and repressed, but once they have been brought into consciousness the energy that has been trapped in repressing them is freed, for more useful, more creative purposes.

Acknowledging and accepting reality means seeing 'the thing as it is'. The fundamental truth for the person with cancer is that his/her reality has suddenly undergone a profound change. This is the case whatever the type of cancer that has been diagnosed – whether it is one of those with a favourable outlook or not, whether it has been discovered at an early stage and is treatable and manageable, or is advanced and likely to be terminal. Whether one is going to die in a month or in a year, or in 40 years, of cancer or of something else, the reality one is facing as a consequence of the diagnosis is the reality of mortality, of death.

This is a huge thing to deal with. It brings with it an onslaught of emotions that for most people are overwhelming: anxiety, terror, anger, grief, despair, fears for one's future and for one's loved ones. These emotions tend to hit all at once, creating an inner upheaval and a commotion within one's heart and head that make it very difficult to think clearly or constructively, or at all. Yoga nidra practice will quiet this commotion down, giving us periods of relative peace that enable us to resume life with our equanimity restored: then we can reflect more calmly on our situation. With regular practice, the effects are cumulative and lasting: our habitual reactions and responses to the situations we face, our ways of being in the world, change. Each time we practise, we learn something about letting go, and this learning stays with us.

Practising yoga nidra creates an inner environment conducive to the transformation of attitudes: in the case of a person confronting a grave illness, the attitude toward the disease and its meaning for his or her life.

A cancer diagnosis is not necessarily a catastrophe. It seems so to almost everyone at first, but many people come to look at it differently: as an opportunity to examine one's life and to change whatever appears to need changing; and as an invitation to heal on a deep level. The illness thus becomes a catalyst for healing, spiritual growth and transformation. If this happens, the entire experience of dealing with the disease and with the treatment, and above all living with the implications of cancer for one's future, becomes a transformative healing process. What at first appeared to be a disaster has become a challenge, even a blessing, and a spur for making constructive changes. The illness comes to be understood, and used, as a stepping-stone to healing and as a path to a richer, more rewarding life. This may lead to the healthy reassessment of priorities on the practical level, such as making significant changes in nutrition, lifestyle, relationships, home life and working life. On a deeper level a profound shift of consciousness may occur, a shift that drives the individual's spiritual journey from that point onwards.

For those who seek its help, yoga will play a significant role in this process. Amongst the many wonderful tools in the 'yoga bag of tools', yoga nidra stands out as a practice of prime importance for anyone going through it.

Now we can look at the four central elements of yoga nidra – sankalpa, the rotation of awareness, the pairs of opposites, and visualization – and at their specific relevance to a person living with cancer, throughout the journey from diagnosis onwards.

Sankalpa

The *sankalpa* is a resolve, a statement of positive intent. It 'works', because it is like a seed planted deep in the rich earth of the subconscious when the mind is quiet and relaxed and ready to absorb it. This seed will germinate, take root, and grow into a healthy plant that will flower and bear fruit, helping us to make the changes we want to make in our life, and to become all that we are capable of being.

Sankalpa directs energy towards healing and spiritual fulfilment: it inspires, supports and sustains the impulse to heal, an impulse not limited to the conscious level. My students with cancer, particularly those who have been practising yoga and yoga nidra for a few years or longer, have experienced and testified to its power; and I, observing this in them and in myself, have come to feel that sankalpa is the heart of yoga nidra.

When we make our sankalpa, we are making a promise to ourselves. We are committing ourselves to both the present and the future: to our task now, and to what we want to do, and be, in the future. Above all, we are asserting our trust that there is a future. People in full health may take the future for granted, but for the newly diagnosed cancer patient who is sure – as so many newly diagnosed people are – that s/he is going to die, the choosing and using of a sankalpa is an affirmative act that opposes this counter-productive, if understandable, fatalism. It is an act of profound significance for healing.

Here is what Swami Satyananda says in *Yoga Nidra* about the role of sankalpa in cancer: "In healing cancer, enormous, sustained endurance and willpower are necessary. In order to attain this, the sankalpa is practised during yoga nidra. The sankalpa is a personal resolution which is released like a seed into the subconscious mind, when the experience of relaxation is deep and the subconscious mind is laid bare and accessible. When this force rises into the sphere of conscious awareness, it can bring about even the impossible in life. Yoga nidra, by maximizing the patient's own conscious efforts to become healthy and whole, is an effective form of cancer therapy."[1]

In *Freedom from the Bondage of Karma*, Swami Rama explains the three kinds of karma: past (the effects of our actions in the past whose consequences we have already experienced); present (the effects of past actions whose consequences we are experiencing in the present); and future, which we are creating by our conscious actions and thoughts in the present. Over the first two kinds of karma we have no control: the actions are done, and we have already experienced their effects, or are experiencing them now, or will experience

276

them in the future. But we can influence the third kind of karma. Swami Rama says, "The arrow which is just now being loaded in our bow is the one which we can control."[2]

So we can think of sankalpa as "the arrow we are just now loading in our bow", a tool with which we can envision and shape the future we want for ourselves, and aim at it. Then our thoughts and actions, directed by sankalpa, can follow the path our arrow cuts for us through the jungle of our fears, insecurities and illusions.

Sankalpa cannot determine the outcome of the healing process, but its contribution to it should not be underestimated. It remains affirmative and significant throughout the journey, even if the cancer becomes terminal. In that final stage, the present becomes infinitely precious, and the future must be differently conceived (but there is still a future).

The rotation of awareness

In the rotation of awareness the body and the mind are brought to a deeply relaxed state. While the focused mind follows the guiding voice around the body, the clamour of painful emotions is calmed, the burden of fear and worry lifted for a time. The act of lightly touching each part of the body with the awareness brings prana, energy, to each part (the awareness is the prana). At the end of the rotation, the awareness is expanded into the whole body, which may then be experienced as filled with energy.

The rotation teaches us to let go. As our attention moves quickly and lightly from each part of the body to the next, not lingering or 'concentrating', we are being taught in the simplest, clearest way not to 'hang on'. The 'letting go' lesson learned during the rotation applies to everything in life: emotions, sensations, experiences, achievements, possessions, disappointments, people. Ultimately, it applies to life itself. Letting go is a lesson for us all to learn. It may be the single most important lesson of yoga nidra, as it arguably is of life.

A person with cancer has a great deal to let go of. All of it is challenging. Much of it has to do with our illusions. We all

277

have illusions, and if we have always been healthy, we probably harbour a couple of particularly tenacious ones.

The illusion of our immortality. We live under this one until we face a life-changing illness. Until then, we probably thought of our time as unlimited. It doesn't seem to matter how old we are when the rude awakening comes: for most, the shattering of the illusion is a shock. But it can be a blessing. For me, acknowledging my mortality at age 58 was liberating. It forced me into the present. It made me acutely conscious of the fact that my time is finite, and I resolved to use the time as well as I could, however long or short it turned out to be. The emotional intensity of that period began to subside during the following year and has long since gone, but the commitment remains, as does the consciousness of finite time.

The illusion that our body is exempt from the ills that visit the bodies of others. In a sense this is part of the mortality illusion, but it has its own special sting, particularly for those who practise and/or teach yoga. We may think: "How could this happen to me? I've practised yoga for years, so how could my body let me down so dramatically?" Others ask us the same question, and their astonishment feeds into our tendency to doubt and blame ourselves. We may scold ourselves, feel guilty, lose trust in our bodies, in ourselves.

But the reality is that all bodies, even the bodies of yogis, and yoga teachers wear out and break down. The great spiritual masters have not been exempt: Bhagavan Sri Ramana Maharishi died of cancer, so did Sri Ramakrishna, among others. Ultimately, the reality is that we are all going to have to let go of life itself, and realizing it now helps prepare for the eventuality. The rotation of awareness in yoga nidra gives us practice in letting go, gently prying us loose from our illusions, and possibly easing our journey towards death.

The rotation of awareness, and yoga nidra as a whole, may also help to renew the person's broken connection with his or her body. A woman who has lost a breast, for example, may feel mutilated, disfigured. She may feel her body has betrayed her by developing cancer, or that it is being irreversibly damaged by chemotherapy or radiotherapy. The re-connection with the body experienced through yoga nidra is nurturing, uplifting and liberating. It opens the way to acceptance, to healing and the return of wholeness.

The pairs of opposites

In the pairs of opposites, as in the rotation of awareness, we move quickly, not lingering, not holding on to comfortable or uncomfortable sensations, or to painful or pleasant emotions, but letting go of each sensation or emotion before proceeding to the next. This part of the practice consolidates the 'letting go' lesson. It teaches us not to get caught up in 'liking' or 'disliking' things. In working with the pairs of opposites we learn that yes, we can let go.

Working with the pairs of opposites sparks our creativity. It teaches us to create, develop, and experience sensations and emotions, and to let go of them. The opposites teach us that sensations and emotions are ephemeral: they come and go, and do not last. Thus this part of the practice helps to release our samskaras, impressions from past experiences.

The opposites teach us detachment, vairagya, the quality that empowers us to stand back a little, not to hold onto sensations and emotions, not to get entangled in them, but to let them come and let them go. We learn to look at what is going on inside us without being afraid of it. We learn that warmth and cold are just warmth and cold, not 'good' and 'bad'. They are just what they are. Pain and pleasure are simply pain and pleasure: we learn to experience them without judging them, without flinching from pain or clinging to pleasure. In creating, developing, feeling, and letting go of sensations and emotions, we learn that sensations and emotions are transitory: they come and they go, and do not last. We learn that 'the thing is as it is'.

For people dealing with a grave illness, and with invasive treatments that generally make them feel worse than the illness itself, this is an exceptionally useful learning. As we work with the opposites, we come to realize that however intense the terror around the diagnosis, however deep the anxiety about the future, however distressing the illness, and however unpleasant or painful the treatment, these sensations and emotions will not last forever. They will end.

Visualization

The different types of visualizations in yoga nidra – rapid images, story lines, the chakras, healing – allow fears and insecurities to surface so that they can be acknowledged, accepted and released. They connect us to our creativity, using our imagination to create and develop images and stories. Working with visualization in yoga nidra, when we are open and sensitive and our imagination can roam freely, helps us to remember and let go of painful stuff from the past. It accesses and releases our samskaras, the impressions grooved into our consciousness by our past experiences. This brings a release from some of the psychological, emotional, and karmic causes of illness and opens us to new experiences.

It is not unusual for people who develop cancer to probe and delve into what they may have done to cause their cancer, or failed to do to avoid it. If they have heard of the concept of karma but lack any real understanding of it, they may conclude "It's my karma", and wonder what they've done to deserve such 'bad' karma. They may be encouraged in this pointless activity by well-meaning friends with a smattering of simplistic New Age knowledge, by the complementary therapists they approach for help, and by misguided fellow yogis. All this is likely to have an entirely negative impact on the healing process.

Karma is surely a factor in the development of a cancer, but there is little to be gained by obsessing over our past sins, whether of commission or omission, since there is nothing we can do on the conscious level to alter our past and unfolding karma. But the release of samskaras in yoga nidra does not happen on the conscious level, so it creates no additional problems and gives us no hang-ups: it just releases the samskaras and the energy held in them. Unlike the guilt-producing, self-scolding and soul-searching, which dissipate energy and block the healing process, it liberates energy and supports the healing process.

Awakening sakshi, developing detachment

Yoga nidra awakens *sakshi*, the witnessing consciousness. Sakshi teaches us detachment, the quality that enables us to stand back a little from what is happening to us, look at it, and observe it accurately.

In one of the dialogues in *The Heart of Yoga*, T.K.V. Desikachar is asked by a student: "Is the ultimate goal of yoga to always be in samadhi?" He replies: "The ultimate goal of yoga is to always observe things accurately".[3]

In *The Power of Now*, Eckhart Tolle says: "Be present as the watcher of your mind – of your thoughts and emotions . . . Don't judge or analyse what you observe. Watch the thought, the emotion, observe your reaction. You will then feel the still, observing presence itself behind the content of your mind, the silent watcher."[4]

The 'observing presence', the 'silent watcher', is sakshi, the witnessing consciousness, through which, when it is awakened, we learn to observe things accurately.

A cancer diagnosis is terrifying. The emotions that arise can be so strong and so intense that one can be overpowered by them and feel incapable of coping with them. The impulse then naturally arises to push them back down, to repress them. Without the help of the practices in the yoga 'bag of tools' it would be easy and natural to give in to that impulse, and to find subterfuges to avoid acknowledging and dealing with the emotions. This is termed 'denial', usually disapprovingly. No one deliberately 'denies' reality unless reality is too painful to bear: sometimes denial is necessary to protect the psyche for a time from truths it is not ready to absorb. But burying emotions for too long traps our energy, and for full healing that energy needs to be released. This is why we need techniques that help us to confront our realities, and to assimilate and accept them.

Through practising yoga nidra we develop our powers of observation. We develop the clarity and the detachment that are needed to confront a diagnosis of cancer, the challenges of invasive treatments, and the uncertainties about the future. We can then step back a little from the emotions it brings in its wake, allow them to arise, look at them clearly, and observe them accurately. When we do this, when we bring them up out of the darkness and shine the light of our awareness – the light of sakshi – on them, they lose their power over us. Then we can face them squarely, acknowledge them, accept them, and eventually let them go – and when that happens, the energy that has been trapped in them is released.

When we are lying still in yoga nidra, following a voice that we trust, allowing ourselves to be guided through the practice, wherever it takes us, we are being given a special kind of strength. Not the brute, 'battling with cancer' strength that we read about in every newspaper obituary, but the deeper strength of acknowledgement and acceptance, the inner strength that enables us to face the challenges we are given and learn their lessons, right through the entire process, and when the time comes, right through to death.

Yoga nidra and the healing journey

When I asked the people in my class at the Yoga Therapy Centre for their thoughts on how yoga nidra has affected them, one young woman, who had been having a difficult time with chemotherapy since she joined the class, said that yoga nidra always gives her a feeling of lightness, of peace, a feeling that a burden has been lifted, and the others all agreed with her.

Another says: "Cancer, like any serious illness, can be seen as an invitation to heal ourselves on a deeper level. Yoga for me has been a very wonderful way to engage in this healing process. Starting in shavasana often feels like coming home into an alive stillness where nothing needs to happen... Ending with yoga nidra offers the forever surprising experience that simple presence with every part of the body creates such restfulness, a sense of being reborn in a different climate."

I will close with the experience of a woman who has been attending the class at the Yoga Therapy Centre since it began eight years ago. At that time she had just finished treatment for an extremely aggressive breast cancer. A few months after joining the class, she wrote: "Not only have I developed my physical and mental strength through the wonderful yoga class of gentle exercises, relaxation and meditation, I have learnt an alternative and holistic way of dealing with the trauma emanating from having had breast cancer. The practice gives me control, hope and peace of mind, as well as a connectedness, within a very supportive and safe environment. No words can really express what a lifeline it has been."

Since then she has been through three recurrences and more intensive chemotherapy and radiotherapy. Her cancer has now recurred again, in her liver, lungs, spine, bones and brain, and is considered terminal. All through these eventful, challenging years she has described yoga as her lifeline; she feels that it has helped her to hold her balance through all the vicissitudes of the past eight years, and to look clearly and unflinchingly at her situation. She has always identified her yoga practice as the grounding, stabilizing influence in her journey, and yoga nidra as the most profoundly healing element in her practice. Now, approaching the end of the journey, she feels that yoga and yoga nidra are helping her towards a healing death.

She says: "Yoga continues to be the core of my being able to deal with this last part of my journey, providing me with deep healing, strength, clarity and peace. My sankalpa has blossomed like a seed deeply planted and forms a guide for my life."

It is a great privilege to pass on the wonderful practice of yoga nidra, and all the other transformative tools of yoga, to people who are in such real and deep need of them. The reward for the teacher is that each of them, in his or her own way, wholeheartedly takes up the tools and uses them on the journey towards wholeness and healing.

References

[1] Saraswati, Swami Satyananda, *Yoga Nidra*, 6th edition, Yoga Publications Trust, Bihar School of Yoga, Munger, Bihar, India, 1998

[2] Rama, Swami, *Freedom from the Bondage of Karma*, Himalayan International Institute of Yoga Science and Philosophy, Honesdale, Pennsylvania, 1977

[3] Desikachar, T.K.V., *The Heart of Yoga: Developing a Personal Practice*, Inner Traditions International, 1995

[4] Tolle, Eckhart, *The Power of Now: A Guide to Spiritual Enlightenment*, Hodder and Stoughton, 2001

References

Chapter 1

[1] Kothari, Manu L. & Mehta, Lopa A., *Living, Dying – A new perspective on the phenomena of disease and dying*, 2nd edn, Other India Press, Goa, India, 1996, pp. 22–23.

Chapter 2

[2] World Health Organization, Manual on Prevention and Control of Common Cancers, 1st edn, World Health Organization Regional Publications, Western Pacific Series No. 20, Authorized reprint by Prentice Hall of India Pvt. Ltd, New Delhi, India, 1998, p. *v*.

[3] World Health Organization, National Cancer Control Programs, World Health Organization, Geneva, 1995, p. 8.

[4] Segerstrom, S, Miller, G. 'Psychological stress and the human immune system: a meta-analytic study of 30 years of inquiry'. *Psychol Bull.* 2004, (4):601–30.

Chapter 3

[5] Garssen, B. 'Psychological factors and cancer development: Evidence after 30 years of research'. *Clinical Psychology Review*, 2004, 24(3):315–338.

[6] Antoni, M.H., Lutgendorf, S.K., Cole, S.W., et al. 'The influence of bio-behavioural factors on tumour biology:

pathways and mechanisms'. *Nature Reviews Cancer* 2006, 6(3):240–248.

Chapter 9

[7] World Health Organization, National Cancer Control Programs, op. cit., p. 42.

[8] World Health Organization, National Cancer Control Programs, op. cit., p. 39–41.

[9] Kaushal, S. P., *Cancer and Herbs*, Vedic Cancer Research Centre, New Delhi, India, 2003

[10] World Health Organization, Manual on Prevention and Control of Common Cancers, op. cit.

Chapter 10

[11] Kothari, Manu L. & Mehta, Lopa A., op. cit. pp. 22–23.

[12] Besant, Annie, *Death – And After*, Theosophical Manual No. 3, 8th edn, The Theosophical Publishing House, Adyar, Madras, India. 1972, pp. 22–23.

[13] Morse, Melvin & Perry, Paul, *Closer to the Light – Learning from the Near-Death Experiences of Children*, Ivy Books, New York, USA, 1991.

Bibliography

Ahuja, M. R., *Cancer: Causes and Prevention*, 1st edn, UBS Publishers' Distributors Ltd, New Delhi, 1997.

Baidyanath Saraswati, N. K. ed, *Voice of Death – Traditional Thoughts and Modern Science*, Bose Memorial Foundation, D. K. Printworld Pvt. Ltd, New Delhi, 2005.

Chinmayananda, Swami, *Kathopanishad – a dialogue with death*, 2nd edn, Central Chinmaya Mission Trust, Mumbai, 1996.

Chinmayananda, Swami, *Shreemad Bhagawad Geeta*, 2nd edn, Chinmaya Publication Trust, Madras, 1961.

Kamath, M. V., *Philosophy of Death and Dying*, Himalayan Institute of Yoga Science & Philosophy, Pennsylvania, USA, 1978.

Moore, Katen & Schmais, Libby, *Living Well with Cancer*, G. P. Putnam's Sons, New York, 2001.

Roitt, Ivan, *Roitt's Essential Immunology*, 9th edn, Blackwell Science Ltd, UK, 1997.

Saraswati, Swami Niranjanananda, *Dharana Darshan*, Yoga Publications Trust, Munger, Bihar, India, 2006.

Saraswati, Swami Niranjanananda, *Yoga Darshan: Vision of the Yoga Upanishads*, Yoga Publications Trust, Munger, Bihar, 2002.

Saraswati, Swami Satyananda, *Asana Pranayama Mudra Bandha*, 4th edn, Yoga Publications Trust, Munger, Bihar, 2008.

Saraswati, Swami Satyananda, *Meditations from the Tantras*, 2nd edn, Yoga Publications Trust, Munger, Bihar, 2000.

Saraswati, Swami Satyananda, *Sure Ways to Self-Realization*, Yoga Publications Trust, Munger, Bihar, 2002.

Saraswati, Swami Satyananda, *A Systematic Course in the Ancient Tantric Techniques of Yoga and Kriya*, Yoga Publications Trust, Munger, Bihar, 2003.

Saraswati, Swami Satyananda, 'The Age of Bhakti'. *Yoga* 11 (1), April 2005.

Saraswati, Swami Satyananda, *Yoga Nidra*, 6th edn, Yoga Publications Trust, Munger, Bihar, 2001.

Saraswati, Swami Sivananda, *The Bhagavad Gita*, 10th edn, The Divine Life Trust Society, Rishikesh, 1998.

Saraswati, Swami Sivananda, *Principal Upanishads*, Divine Life Society, Shivanandanagar, U.P., India, 1993.

Samarpan: Living the Divine Connection, from the teachings of Swami Sivananda Saraswati and Swami Satyananda Saraswati, Yoga Publications Trust, Munger, Bihar 2008.

Upasana: In the Presence of the Divine, from the teachings of Swami Sivananda Saraswati and Swami Satyananda Saraswati, Yoga Publications Trust, Munger, Bihar 2007.

Index of Practices